Self Help Book For

Nail Biting

Adults

"Mind Over Matter"

By

Asanka S. Jayarathne

The IT Guy Who Cured Nail Biting Habit

Dedication

To my unseen mentor and the best teacher in my life.

MR.BOB PROCTOR

Last But Not Least To My Best Buddies,

My Loving Mom & Dad

SUSILA & WIJESIRI

Table of Contents

This is where we connect…

Thank you for choosing to buy this book! I am thrilled to have you as a reader and I am confident that this book will exceed your expectations. You have my personal guarantee that you won't be disappointed, and you'll feel proud of your purchase decision.

Please, leave an honest review…

However, even if it seems overwhelming right now, there is something you can do to help me. Online reviews are vital to the success of any product or service in the current digital era, and my book is no exception. You can help me reach a wider audience and encourage those who struggle with nail biting to find this game-changing book by posting a review on the site where you bought it.Let me explain why your review is so crucial. Online platforms rank products based on the number of reviews and their positivity. This means that the more reviews and positive feedback a product has, the more visible it will be to a wider audience. By sharing your honest thoughts and feedback about my book, you'll be helping me to reach more people who may benefit from its content.

But, it's not just about me. The law of reciprocity says that by helping others, we help ourselves too. By leaving a review,

1. you'll be helping future readers to make an informed decision about whether or not this book is right for them.

2. You'll feel great knowing that you've played a part in helping others those who suffer nail-biting.

3. So, I'm asking you to please take a moment to leave an honest review of this book after you've read it. Your review will make all the difference in helping this book to succeed, and I truly appreciate your support. Thank you!

I will make it very easy for you, after you read this book, just scan the below QR code and it will take you where you need to leave a review. All you need to do is log in and write your honest review about my book.

To be honest and fair to you, I constantly adjust the price of my e-book, but I have one more thing I want you to know before reading this book in any format. My print book's price may never change. You might even be a lucky duck and have received this for free, or you might have paid up to $9.99. However, I want you to know that regardless of the cost of the e-book you purchased, This book's "used value" and the time and work it took to organize everything chronologically and share the techniques I personally utilized to "cure" my nail-biting for good, as well as the turning point this book is making in your life, assure you it is worth a whole lot of money!

If you've made it this far, I want you to know that you're not alone. As someone who struggled with nail biting for over 35 years, I know exactly what you're going through. The constant urge to bite your nails can be overwhelming, and it's easy to feel trapped in a cycle that's hard to break.
But I'm here to tell you that there is hope. I've been in your shoes, and I've found a way out. And now, I want to help you do the same.

Together, we'll embark on a journey that will transform your life. You'll learn how to break the habit of nail biting, once and for all. You'll discover the tools and techniques that I used to overcome this challenge, and you'll see firsthand how they can work for you too.

" I'm not promising that this journey will be easy,
but I can promise you that it will be worth it. "

Imagine feeling confident and proud of your hands for the first time in years. Imagine being able to shake hands with someone without feeling ashamed.

This journey can give you all of that, and more.

" And ladies, you can now go crazy with your nail art."

So, if you're ready to take the first step towards a new life, I'm here to help you. Let's do this together, and let's make sure that nail biting is a thing of the past.

Think outside the box

I have another big favor to ask of you - the most important one yet!

As you embark on this journey to cure your nail-biting habit, I urge you to approach this book with an open and unbiased mind. You've already invested in it, and now it's time to fully commit to the process of change.

"If you are NOT open-minded and NOT ready to adopt some tiny changes and commitments to your daily routine for the next month, unfortunately, this could be another "self-help" book written by some "self-help guru" that ends up stacking on your book shelf!"

Throughout this book, I may reference certain individuals or stories to help illustrate my points. particularly Mr.Bob Proctor, and you will understand why!

But rest assured, I will do my best to keep things fun, engaging, and interactive. This is not your typical, boring self-help book.

Rather, it's a personal journey filled with tips and tricks that helped me cure my own nail-biting habit in just two short weeks (that's for me as a severe nail biter!)—and you're free to try them for yourself!

Remember, this is your journey and yours alone. You don't need anyone else by your side to make it happen. All you need is yourself and this book. As you read on, you'll begin to understand why thinking inside-out is the key to overcoming negative habits and beliefs. So keep an open mind and get ready to transform your life. You won't regret it.

Think

> *"Two percent of the people think; three percent of the people think they think; and ninety-five percent of the people would rather die than think."*
>
> — *George Bernard Shaw*

Do you ever feel like you're just going through the motions of life, without really stopping to think about your choices or actions? Well, according to the famous playwright George Bernard Shaw, you're not alone. In fact, he suggests that a shocking 95% of people would rather avoid thinking altogether, even if it means missing out on growth and success. Only a small fraction of people, just 2%, actually engage in genuine critical thinking, while another 3% believe they do. This perspective is truly alarming, and it begs the question: are we really living our lives to the fullest if we're not taking the time to think about what we're doing?

Shaw's quote serves as a powerful reminder that thinking is a valuable and necessary tool for success and fulfillment. By making a conscious effort to incorporate critical thinking into our daily lives, we can join the ranks of the small percentage of individuals who are truly thriving. So, let's take a moment to pause and reflect, and start living more intentional, thoughtful lives today.

Are you ready to take control of your life and start living intentionally? It's time to start thinking, and not just any kind of thinking - critical thinking.

From the age of sixteen and beyond, it's important to ask yourself three fundamental questions every single day:

1. Who are you?
2. What are you doing?
3. And where are you going in life?

By taking the time to reflect on these questions and write down your answers with a pen and a piece of paper, you can start to gain clarity and direction in your life. And let me be clear - you don't need any gimmicky nail-biter products or any other trendy items to succeed.
I won't be promoting anything that isn't necessary for your personal growth and success. It's time to focus on what truly matters and start using the tools that are already at your disposal - your own thoughts and the power of critical thinking.

" What really matters is you, and your thinking here. Not nail biting "

So, are you ready to think this way and start this journey with me?

Let's get real for a moment, shall we? I'm guessing if you're reading this, you've probably tried everything under the sun to stop your nail-biting habit. And let's be honest, nothing has worked so far, right? Well, don't worry, my friend, because I was in the same boat as you not too long ago.

Now, if young adult like me, I'm sure you've spent hours upon hours searching for a solution on YouTube, Google, or wherever else you could find. But alas, still no luck! But hey, that's why you've got me and this book. We're gonna tackle this thing head-on, and I promise you, by the time you're done reading, you'll have kicked that nasty habit to the curb. And if you're a youngster, well, first of all, kudos to you for being proactive about breaking this habit early on! But seriously, what are you doing here? Just kidding, you're in the right place too. We're gonna work together and make sure you never have to worry about nail-biting again.

So let's think outside the box, people! Let's take control of our habits and our lives.

And let's have some fun while we're at it!

Oh, one more thing! please read the following few tricks and tips that will help you thinking before start,

Thinking Inside – Out

Do you ever feel like you're stuck in a cycle of negative beliefs and feelings? Maybe you constantly tell yourself that you're not good enough, or that you'll never be successful. These negative thoughts can quickly become a habit, leading to a self-perpetuating cycle of negativity that's hard to break free from. But there is a way to change your thought patterns and start living a more positive, fulfilling life. It's time to start thinking inside-out.

Thinking inside-out means taking a step back from your negative thoughts and examining them from a different perspective. Instead of letting them control you, you can learn to control them.

By understanding that your thoughts and feelings are not necessarily reflective of reality, you can start to shift your mindset in a more positive direction. But in order to do so, you need to be willing to learn something new.

Feeding your mind with new, positive ideas is essential for breaking the cycle of negative thoughts. This could mean reading books on personal development, listening to motivational podcasts, or surrounding yourself with positive, uplifting people. By filling your mind with new ideas and beliefs, you can start to rewire your brain to think in a more positive way.

But changing your thought patterns is not an overnight process. It takes time, effort, and a commitment to making positive changes in your life.

It's important to be patient with yourself and to practice self-compassion along the way. You may experience setbacks or negative thoughts, but remember that these are all part of the process. The key is to keep moving forward, one step at a time.

In addition to feeding your mind with positive ideas, it's also important to take care of your physical health. Exercise, healthy eating, and getting enough sleep can all have a positive impact on your mental wellbeing. By taking care of your body, you can improve your mood, boost your energy levels, and feel more confident in yourself.

Thinking inside-out is not just about changing your thoughts, but also about changing your actions. If you want to see positive changes in your life, you need to take action towards your goals.

This could mean setting small, achievable goals for yourself and celebrating each milestone along the way. By taking consistent action towards your goals, you can build momentum and start to see real progress in your life.

In conclusion, if you're struggling with negative beliefs and feelings, it's time to start thinking inside-out. By understanding that your thoughts and feelings are not necessarily reflective of reality, and by feeding your mind with new, positive ideas, you can start to shift your mindset in a more positive direction. Remember to be patient with yourself, take care of your physical health, and take consistent action towards your goals. With time and effort, you can break free from the cycle of negativity and start living a more positive, fulfilling life.

I haven't even got started yet, Let's dive-in then…

Are you ready to unlock the full potential of this book and transform your life?

Here are some tips to get you started:

1. First, make it a habit to read at least one chapter from Chapter 05 every day for the next month. Trust me, you'll know the day when you no longer need to do this daily.

2. Next, don't skip the exercises and affirmations explained in Chapter 05. They're designed to help you put the concepts into action and reinforce positive changes in your life.

3. Finally, keep an open mind and a positive attitude. The transformative power of this book lies in your willingness to embrace new ideas and make real changes.

So, are you ready to take the first step towards a better life? Let's get started!

PREFACE

Scorching sun makes temperatures now here in Qatar over 110 degrees towards the evening. But, this is the summer of July 2019 and everybody should remain inside; there is even a standard from the legislature that nobody should work from 11.00 AM to 3.30 PM outside. On the off chance that you get found doing any work during this time, you are in trouble! Period! Not just you! But the company you are working for. It's that hot!

Keeping aside the climate from where I live, my name is Asanka Jayarathne. I was brought up in the most beautiful Island nation, Sri Lanka. I am 36 years old as I write this book. There is generally nothing special about me, I am a normal person just like you! An IT Guy; passing my youth by and thinking of becoming rich one day like everybody else, purchasing fancy cars, homes, to have more hair than I have and to maybe lose a couple of pounds. I have simple needs like any another person. Keeping aside my fantasies and keeping in mind that I am chasing them, there is one dream as of late that has worked out as expected, and I am going to tell you what it is; I've defeated an awful stinky habit! BITING NAILS!!

As of now, I have done it as explained in this book. I needed to share this thought since I know how it feels, how urgent the change is and how you blame your experiences and the amount you endure with this habit.

The individuals who hotshot in television shows, the individuals who compose books or articles about nail-biting, may never have had this habit in their life. So they express their thoughts on their perspective and knowledge but not with their daily life. Well, I don't blame them. They are also trying to help you too!

This book that I have made for you incorporates every one of my encounters, the activity plan, and you can rest assured that I accomplished my habit and conquered it. So these substances are not theoretical. These that I am presenting to you, all are interactive and they all work.

Understand me well! I have been there for over 30 years, technically my entire childhood and my young life endured with this habit, so I know how agonizing, liable and terrible this habit is.

I need my dear readers to comprehend and know about the habit from here through this book, and I urge you to do some research of the habit that you are a victim of. Give me a chance to begin here.

"KEEP THIS BOOK WITH YOU AS A MANUAL FOR THE FINISH OF THIS HABIT FOR THE LAST TIME."

Researches state that a habit of nail-biting has no definite reason for how it begins, other than it is a habit that is gradually created as we bite our fingers and nails to relieve our stress. In the concerned part, researchers state that nail-biting is another indication of OCD (Obsessive Compulsive Disorder) as they explain this is additionally, an impulsive habit. The individual knows about the habit, and can't deliberately stop it.

You may find out about OCD and get a thought. As you read, you will comprehend, as indicated by your behavior, whether you feel you are OCD or not. If you have ever perceived yourself having OCD, be straightforward with yourself and go for treatment as soon as you can.

This book is especially composed without anyone else's input and with NO formal training of psychology (By calling, I am an IT Systems & Network Administrator). However, with my readings and experiences alongside my workforce venture, what this book suggests does work.

THIS BOOK IS FAR FROM FOCUSED ON ANY OTHER PRACTICES OR MENTAL CIRCUMSTANCES AND SHOULD NOT BE RECOMMENDED TO ANYONE WITH OTHER MENTAL DISORDERS. LET THE PHYSCOLOGITS DO THEIR WORK ON THEM.

As shown in later sections, this strategy isn't a remedy that utilizing anything. No items need to be used and no other individual needs to participate with you through the procedure. This is you who is making a committed decision, to beat the habit, with awareness through knowledge and a few little exercises. It's quite an exciting journey, but that's it! Nothing fancy here!

Every one of the procedures I have used here, is from the lessons I have learned and read from Mr. Bob Proctor, especially about the Law of Polarity and the Law of Vibration. Furthermore, some of the information I have accumulated through readings about the subconscious mind.

Also personal growth books like; *Napoleon Hill's Think And Grow Rich, Psycho-Cybernetics by Dr.Maxwell Maltz, The Power of Subconscious Mind by Dr.Joseph Murphy, Bob Proctors' You Were Born Rich,* Etc.

(I strongly recommend for you all to obtain an eBook or hardcover of the above books and start reading right away!)

DISCLAIMER

AS YOU HAVE ALL SEEN IN THE BOOK DESCRIPTION, THIS BOOK IS NOT FOR THOSE WHO BLAME THE WORLD FOR THEIR OWN PROBLEMS; DECEIVING THEMSELVES WITH PRODUCTS ON THE MARKET THAT ARE MOSTLY NOT GOING TO WORK AT ALL. PEOPLE WHO ARE PESSIMESTIC, LAZY AND MOST IMPORTANTLY...

"NOT GOING TO DO THE EXERCISES I AM EXPLAINING HERE"

AND YOU HAVE BEEN WARNED THROUGH THE DESCRIPTION ABOUT THIS BOOK AND I AM SORRY IF YOU BOUGHT THIS BOOK FOR NOTHING!

IF YOU ARE NOT THAT PERSON, BUCKLE UP AND I WILL PROMISE YOU THIS LITTLE BOOK IS WORTH A WHOLE LOT MORE THAN THE FEW BUCKS YOU HAVE SPENT ALREADY!

Let's be honest here, no matter what you think about yourself, rich, poor, accomplished, so on and on, a nail-biting habit makes us inferior from others; despite it just being a habit with cosmetics concerns (for the most part). We bite our nails in the general public, like in the work place, with or without our knowledge! Imagine when you are biting your nails, it seems as though you are biting your fingers! Try not to be embarrassed! Be that as it may, it is true!

Something critical to understand is that we are constantly fueling this habit when we could have halted long back, we are less mindful about it. We should confront it. We have to comprehend where we are and what we are doing. Along these lines, we have to find out about this habit. We are going to start from somewhere and stop it anyway! How? I will show to you how through this book.

Something About Chapters

The initial four chapters will give you a background to understand more about nail-biting, so you might call it scratching the surface or boring! That's OK! But do you know something?

Straightaway, if you are feeling "lazy" and begin thinking that you purchased this book to dispose of nail-biting, so let us just come to the heart of the matter! Or if you feel that it will bore you to go through the initial four chapters, then I will give you a chance to skip them! I have written this book that way, so you can begin directly from chapter number five if you so wish. It clarifies my well-ordered encounters and techniques that I used to conquer the habit.

I guarantee that it will enable you to progress much further!

I have composed this when I have spare time in my office.IT folks don't work routinely as you are probably are aware! We work on demand. So, it is obvious that we are have a lot of spare time some days. I am blessed. What's more, it took longer than I thought to complete this, and to set it up in a language for everyone to get it. I believe this will be the last resource (this book) that you need to stop this habit, and I want you to enjoy all that life has to offer. All the best to your committed decision.

"SETTLE ON A COMMITTED DECISION THAT YOU WILL STOP NAIL-BITING AND START READING..."

Wishing you all peace and success!

Asanka Jayarathne

From Doha (State of Qatar)

asankajayarathne@hotmail.com

CHAPTER ONE

Ex Nail-Biter Me!

I was biting my nails for as far back as I can recollect, I don't know the time from when I first began this habit. Yet if somebody approached me and asked me what I had done about it and so on; I would say, I went for treatment, I googled it, I watched YouTube recordings, I tried rubber bands hurting my skin, chewing gums to divert my triggers, etc.

Be that as it may, I didn't find my solution. If you took a look at my nails, you would have seen how much of an obsessive nail biter I was. A large portion of my google search and other research was wound up with products on the market that I needed to have a go at, burning through many dollars.

The fact that you should spend, time and time again, hundreds or maybe thousands of dollars, on the off chance that you will find a successful treatment. It doesn't give any real assurance (I tried it, I effectively burned through cash, and I know it for a fact).

I'm completely aware of the psych behind a nail biter, as I have experienced it fully, for almost all of my childhood and my youth until the early in 2019.

Despite how badly and seriously we need to overcome this habit, we still bite our nails.

We are not alone people. There is at least 30 percent of the world's population who are suffering from this. I used the word "suffer" here because I did suffer. No matter what other "non nail biters' think, it's no joke here folks, we are suffering people!

The more awful part is the "guilty feeling" during and after biting our nails. I realized how disturbed and helpless the feeling was when taking a peek sometimes at those destroyed nails and cuticles, thinking multiple times and promising to yourself that you will never do it again. Only to start it again just 30 minutes later. Is it worth the pain when your nails and cuticles get infected, or when you can't open a lid off a bottle as a result of no nails, and the skin is so fragile that we can't do anything that individuals having pleasant nails could do.

Another enemy is the battle between the guilty feeling and nail-biting. That makes us more frustrated and even further discouraged with our lives, and the feeling is hopeless! We take peek at other's wonderful fingers and nails, hate ourselves and even often feel inferior. The torment, the blood, and the worst nightmare of it all - cuticle infections!

Listen! I have a piece of news for you. A generally excellent one. I ceased it completely! I could stop it without hurting myself. Indeed, even without pinching myself, without spending a dollar! I am never again a nail biter. I have conquered the habit.

What's more, I'm going to disclose to you how I did it.

In this book, I am going to take a typical heavy nail-biter, who began to read this book's procedure, and divide the process into three categories. These stages are explained as chapters for your convenience.

- The Initial Stage (THE energizing STAGE)
- The Interim (CHALLENGING TIME)
- The Final last Stage (AFTER RESULTS)

NOTE

From here on, as explained, if you like to come to the heart of the matter of my ways, you may avoid the initial four chapters and begin reading from chapter five. But I'm seriously recommending that you read all of the chapters from the beginning and understand the expectations that could support your life. As you are a chronic nail biter, you need to be mindful that there are different issues related to nail-biting. So, you have some issues to deal with. Not just biting nails. As a matter of fact, the most important and the most significant thing is "YOU NEED TO ACCEPT AND UNDERSTAND THAT YOU ARE A PATHOLOGICAL NAILBITER ". Only from this point, can we begin.

Every nail-biter has a dream. I had that dream. The dream in having beautiful healthy nails.

Why Do We Bite Our Nails?

Let me tell you about one of my personal experiences. "Why are you biting your nails you idiot?" - I remember one of my best buddies asked me 15 years back.

Of course, he didn't say it because he was mad at me. He was concerned. We were office colleagues working together at the same institute and we used to go for some swimming lessons. He yelled at me because I was biting my nails in the pool.

Who is that stressed out that they have to bite their nails in the pool? Weird, right?

Nail-Biting always went along with my emotions. Let me explain with examples.

- Something happened quickly that made me concerned (This counts for when I was watching a nice movie and something tense would happen next)

- When I was feeling bored

- When I felt like I needed a snack

Biting off my nails gave me a very nice stimulation, feeling of satisfaction. It made me feel okay! Just like people need to smoke.

Other triggers:

- When I felt a hangnail appear on another finger.
- When I felt skin growing around my nails.
- When I checked to see if there were any getting too long.

The disaster was after I bit my nails and the pain started. I ruined my nails, fingers and the skin; even hurting myself in the process, sometimes creating a wound! Whatever grown nails there were, would disappear! Blood came out. It hurt! Then where was my fun?

It had gone. I felt, miserable! Sound familiar? I had a whole 30 years of this...

Listen, there is no one to help you with this. It is you and only you who has to confront this and find a solution to the matter. This book is the correct one.

It is not funny when you having infections.

I remember my parents shouting at me so many times, my father slapped me for this, and I was humiliated in the middle of a crowd. You know the sad part was also my younger sister and brother were also biting their nails. I guess they followed me because I am their big brother.

I had this issue since I could remember, until the rising year of 2019, until I understood this method. So, if I do the math, it's some 30 years!

I still have the physical damage caused by nail-biting, and thank God there are no longer social impacts. Some nail-biters tend to bite selected fingers to maintain a balance between the habit and the nails.

What about me? I used to bite all of them equally, so there was no exception for my fingers to look dirty, unhealthy and ugly. Plus, I suffered with occasional infections such as Paronychia where my nails became severely deformed. In addition to this, it even it made some of my teeth crooked. Thank you nail-biting!

You may read some articles about health and social impacts alongside with this book, so you can give an extra push against your habit with the added understanding about what is going on with you! I can't stress enough about the awareness of the habit. That's why you should read this book. Just gain some more knowledge.

I know the habit caused me a lack of quality of life, shameful feelings, guilty feelings and this is how.

You're doing the right thing. You've now acknowledged that you have a nail biting problem and now you're on the road to fixing it. Good job!

I'm actually going to help you a lot in this book, because I'm going to tell you about a few of the little known side effects that biting your nails can cause.

And when you hear about them, you'll certainly think twice about biting your nails again! (This is not the solution though. That comes from chapter five)

Okay, so we all know that biting your nails is an unsightly habit. Afterwards, your nails are all crooked and the skin underneath is red and damaged.

But did you know, that if you bite your nails chronically, then you are five times more likely to get an infection in your hands? Now, to give you some idea, most infections are harmless; but some are really harmfull. I heard once about a man, who's arm becomes infected whilst out fishing. Fast forward 24 hours, and doctors were fighting to save his arm. Pretty dramatic, I know, but that was one of the results of an infection!

Whilst the odds are in your favor that you probably won't lose your arm, the odds aren't so good about you damaging your gums. If you're chewing your nails 50 times a day, then your gums are getting a lot of raw treatment up there in your mouth. So much so, that they can become damaged quite severely and even cause teeth displacement for years. Look up gingival injury on Google and check out some of the pictures - really not nice!

This is the worst of the lot - you could allow bacteria to pass into your body - most notably pinworms that live inside of you and multiply by feeding off food from your intestines. Again, pretty unlikely to happen to you - but not unheard of!

There's nothing more annoying than a habit that you just can't kick. It can be so frustrating because it's ingrained in your head so badly, that you just do it subconsciously without even thinking about it.

I know what it is like for chronic nail biters. I've been trying to kick one of my other chronic habits recently; I always say "like" in my sentences. He "like" went out and it was "like" really frustrating 'cos "like"... And so on - you get the idea.So many people must have a bad first impression of me. Recently, I've managed to lose that habit so I'm pretty pleased.

Back to the subject, I've found what has got to be the best cure for nail biters out there. It's an ingenious way of stopping you bite your nails - and it's so easy!

You see, the problem with biting your nails as mentioned earlier, is that you can end up with infections, gum problems, misaligned teeth and even in the most serious cases, pinworms that live in your intestines and feed off of your food. Yes, I'm not joking - all the aforementioned problems have been caused by chronic nail biters in the past!

CHAPTER TWO

My Life After I Watched the Movie "The Secret"

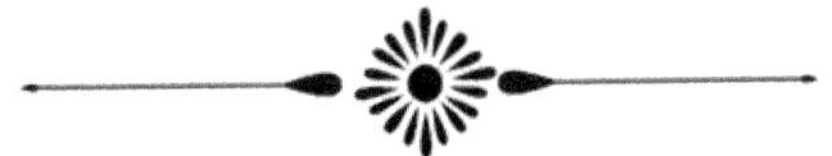

First Time I Watched It!

I still remember the first time I watched the movie Secret in August 2016. It was a short video clip on Facebook subtitled in Sinhalese (My mother tongue), so I just checked it out thinking it would be like just another self-help movie, until Bob Proctor asked that question.

What Do You Really Want?

There were stars who already understood the secret like, Dr. Joe Vitale, John Assaraf, Loral Langemeier, Marie Diamond, Rev. Dr. Michael Beck with, Esther Hicks, Bill Harris, Jack Canfield, Bob Doyle, Mike Dooley, Fred Alan, John Hagelin, Neale Donald Walsh, Dr. John F.Demartini, Marci Shimoff, Dr. John Hagelin. I say a big thanks to all of them for helping me understand what they shared in the movie "Secret".

Bob appeared in the first few minutes in the video when he asked, "What do you want?" That question, it took all my attention because no one has ever asked me something like that in my whole life. Not even my parents! Has anyone asked that question to you? Probably the day before when your parents want to buy you a birthday gift.

"Just take a piece of paper, write it down!" That's what Bob said.

I was so skeptical. Is that going to give me what I want? So, I watched it until the end. Then I thought, this is really something and I wanted to find the full video, so I found it. Watched again, again and again! What they were talking about spoke frequencies! Vibrations. If you hold a thought in your mind, how it would manifest to physical or monetary equivalents?

I don't know the exact reason, but these things started to make me curious, and I wanted to learn more and more about this stuff.

I was always curious about the law of attraction. I have heard of it before, even tried it using visualization which those gurus teach on the internet. Didn't work for me though. Even before I watched and read so many videos and articles; none of them got my attention like the "movie Secret".

All of the characters in the movie are successful people, in which general people considered them to have achieved something extraordinary. They are rich. Maybe not so much with money. Their faces are glowing with wonderful vibes, they always have a smile on their faces. They are not fake. Period!

Someone might take at a glance at "The Secret", and think it is being partial and only talking about "The Law of Attraction", but there are deep concepts behind it. First of all, if you have listened to Bob Proctor, he always says, "you must first study the 'Law of Vibration' before you study the concept 'The Law Of Attraction'. You must at least have to have a foundation understanding of what these are if you want to get use out of them."

> "WE ALL WORK WITH ONE INFINITE POWER. WE ALL GUIDE OURSELVES BY THE SAME LAWS"
> *BOB PROCTOR*

Bob Proctor once said, "We all work with one infinite power." We all guide ourselves by the same laws." But what exactly are these laws? In simple terms, these are the universal principles that govern everything in our world. And just because we can't always see or understand them doesn't mean they don't exist.

Take electricity, for example. You can't physically see it, but you know how useful it is in your everyday life. So, you have no doubt that it exists. Similarly, there are other things in the universe that we can't see, but that doesn't mean they're not there.

In fact, "The Secret" explains how understanding and harnessing these universal laws can help us achieve success and happiness in our lives. So don't let your inability to see or comprehend these laws hold you back from unlocking their full potential.

By embracing them, you can tap into the power of the universe and achieve anything you desire.

Dr. Wernher Von Braun, a pioneering force behind the space program, expressed a profound realization about the universe. He marveled at the incredible precision and order of the natural laws that govern the cosmos, leading him to conclude that something like divine will must have played a role in the creation of the universe.

These laws are so precise that we are able to build a spaceship and travel to the moon, calculating the exact timing of the journey to the fraction of a second. These same natural laws that enable us to explore the vastness of space also affect our daily lives in countless ways. It's amazing to think that everything around us, from the rising sun to the changing seasons, is guided by the intricate workings of these laws. By understanding and working in harmony with these laws, we can unlock our full potential and achieve incredible things in our own lives."

Let me tell you about one of the most powerful laws in the universe: the Law of Vibration. This law states that everything in the universe, including our own bodies, is in a constant state of vibration based on our thoughts and emotions. Yes, you heard that right! Every single thought and emotion we have creates a unique vibration within us.

Now, you might be wondering, How does this apply to nail-biting? Well, the Law of Vibration plays a crucial role in overcoming any habit, and that includes the habit of nail-biting. By understanding the correct vibrations to emit, we can train our minds to break free from the negative thought patterns that keep us stuck in our habits.

But hold on, there's more! The Law of Vibration is closely tied to the Law of Attraction, which is another essential law we'll be exploring later in this book. In fact, understanding the Law of Vibration is the first step to mastering the Law of Attraction and attracting positive changes into our lives.

"So, let's dive deeper into the Law of Vibration and start harnessing its power to overcome nail-biting and transform our lives for the better!"

Are you curious about the law of attraction? This powerful law is based on the Law of Vibration, which states that everything in the universe is in constant motion, including our thoughts and emotions. Our brains act as the central switching station for our bodies vibrations, meaning that our thoughts and feelings directly impact the frequency at which our bodies vibrate.

But how does the Law of Attraction actually work? It's simple: when we focus our thoughts on positive, productive, and joyful things, our bodies vibrate at a similar frequency, attracting more of the same from the universe. On the other hand, negative and destructive thoughts can lead to negative outcomes.

To truly grasp the power of the Law of Attraction, it's important to study its relationship to the Law of Vibration. So, I highly recommend diving deeper into this fascinating topic to unlock the full potential of your thoughts and emotions. Get ready to harness the power of the universe and manifest the life you desire.

The Law Of Cause And Effect

The Law of Cause and Effect is one of the fundamental laws of the universe, and it applies to everything we do. This is not only true for our actions, but it also applies to our thoughts and emotions. In fact, it is so universal that many religions and philosophies, such as Buddhism, are built upon this law. So, what does the Law of Cause and Effect mean for us and our bad habits? Simply put, it means that every action we take or thought we have has a consequence. If we consistently engage in negative actions or thoughts, we will experience negative consequences in our lives. On the other hand, if we consistently engage in positive actions or thoughts, we will experience positive consequences.

But how can we use this law to overcome our bad habits? The key is to identify the root cause of the habit and take action to change it. For example, if we have a habit of nail-biting, the root cause might be anxiety or stress. By addressing and reducing our anxiety or stress, we can change the cause and, therefore, the effect (the habit of nail-biting).

It is important to note that the law of cause and effect is not just applicable to our bad habits. It applies to all areas of our lives, including our relationships, careers, and health. By being mindful of the actions and thoughts we engage in and understanding the consequences they have, we can make more intentional choices that lead to positive outcomes.

In conclusion, the law of cause and effect is a powerful tool we can use to transform our lives. By understanding that every action, thought, and emotion has a consequence, we can make intentional choices that lead to positive outcomes.

So, take a moment to reflect on your habits and the causes behind them. What actions can you take today to change the cause and create a positive effect?

The Law Of Polarity

The Law of Polarity is the cornerstone of my book and the key to unlocking a happier, more fulfilling life. This powerful force dictates that everything in the universe has an opposite, and by focusing on the positive, we can transform the negative aspects of our lives.

In fact, most of the book is dedicated to applying the law of polarity to overcome bad habits, such as nail-biting. By creating a new model that is the exact opposite of the habit, we can render the old behavior obsolete. This means focusing on positive actions, such as self-care and meditation, instead of negative ones like nail-biting.

But the law of polarity is not just about overcoming bad habits. By applying it to our lives, we can shift our perspective and start seeing the world in a new light. We can focus on the good things that are happening rather than dwelling on the bad. This shift in mindset can have a profound impact on our mental health and wellbeing, helping us to overcome negative thought patterns and behaviors.

It's important to note that the law of polarity is not about denying negative emotions or experiences. Rather, it's about acknowledging them and then focusing on the positive aspects of our lives. By doing so, we can create a sense of balance and harmony that allows us to move forward with confidence and joy.

So, if you're looking to transform your life, I urge you to give the law of polarity a try. Focus on the positive, and watch as your life begins to transform before your eyes. It's an incredible journey, and one that you won't regret.

After watching the movie, again and again, I came to understand that, just like the law of gravity, there are other laws we are under in this universe.
We are all the same children of the universe under one infinite power and we are under and guided by all laws in the universe, whether you like or not, believe it or not.

What Are These Laws? I Will Explain A Few.

If you can't see or understand something, that doesn't mean it doesn't exist. As of "The Secret ", Bob Proctor gives a nice and handy example, electricity. Can you see it? You know how useful electricity is in our life. So, you do believe that electricity exists, right? Even if you can't see it. What about other things in this universe you can't see that you may or may not know exist?

1. How about the law of gravity?

You know it exists. But you know you can't see it. You know that if you release anything heavier than the air, it will fall. Why? Because of the law of gravity. Nothing else. Why we are circling the sun? Why is our moon circling our earth? You know why. You learnt it in your junior schools. If someone tells you that the law of gravity doesn't exist, for sure your face will have a dumbfounded look. Right?

We all are guided by some laws that exist in this universe whether you know about it, or believe it or not! Here are a few more, including the two laws that we apply and use in this book.

2. Law of Vibration

This is one of the most important laws, and in this book we use this law to overcome the nail-biting habit. According to the law of vibration, everything moves. Our whole body is in constant vibrations according to the thought patterns we have. Nothing rests. In later chapters, we are going to learn and use correct vibrations to get rid of the habit.

This is the core concept we need to understand and apply change to our habit patterns (paradigms) and we need to understand the law of vibration before learning about the law of attraction.

3. Law of Attraction

According to the law of vibration, our whole molecular structure vibrates... nothing rests. Our brain, which is considered as the central switching station, is the main part of vibration in our body according to our thought frequencies.

This you will not understand fully until you read some contents related to the topic. So, I strongly ask you to go through materials about the relationship of the law of vibration and the law of attraction.

So, how does this law of attraction work? Our body is vibrating to the frequency according to what we are thinking of, as we are thinking more often about something productive, positive and being happy all the time, our body also vibrates similar to those frequencies which attract the same from the universe. What could happen if someone always carried hate, envy, fear, or any other destructive thoughts? You guessed it, bad things. That's why this is so important.

NOTE

You need to understand these concepts with feelings, emotions and from your heart. Just by reading any book by heart will not make any sense unless you understand core concepts of it.

EXAMPLE:

If you want to be a success, you need to always have a positive attitude with "how to be successful" thoughts, that help you feel and believe that you have already acquired success in your life.

There are NO shortcuts to understand these, nor short paths that you will become a success. You have to have productive thoughts more often, and bring sudden hunches coming to you for action with desire and faith. along with organized planning.

There are 13 principles of success that Napoleon Hill explains in his *"Think And Grow Rich"* book and I have only taken a few of them here.

Remember, nothing will work for you if you don't take any "Action". Unless you take action to achieve anything you want, the action is followed by an investment with your time, money or any other compensation for the people you seek help from in order to achieve your target. Read this book if you want to succeed, don't try to be perfect with everything. Just take action according to the plan explained in here.

- While you are biting your nails, you are thinking about it. Consciously feeling guilty but subconsciously feeling satisfied. This is a clash causes you to feel stressed out.

- While you are biting your nails, it looks ugly and unprofessional. Not only that, when you are in an open discussion or meeting, you tend to hide your hands worrying that others might notice your busted nails. I know this feeling.

- When you are sitting with your boss, in an interview presentation, you tend to hide your fingers.

Let me explain to you what kind of person I was before watching the movie Secret in the next chapter.

CHAPTER THREE

Learning Pace For 3 Years

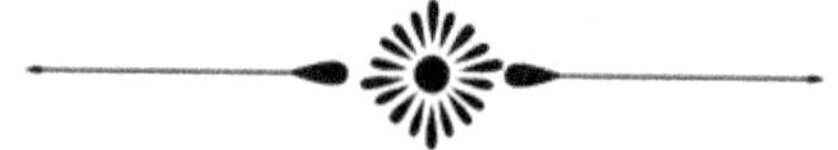

How I Learned What I Learned

Through the teachings of Mr. Bob Proctor, I was so curious about the subconscious mind and how it impacts our lives. I continued watching his recordings and purchased a couple of books which made me think about the human mind, particularly the subconscious mind.

My life was so natural after that. I have unwittingly changed how I figure, how I should hold positive thoughts; all an opportunity to show beneficial things in the event that I truly need them.

I began to read daily "The Power Of Subconscious Mind " by Dr.Joseph Murphy and "Think And Grow Rich " by Napoleon Hill, "You Were Born Rich" by Bob Proctor, "Thoughts Are Things" by Bob Proctor and Greg S. Reid. Regardless of how much I grasp those concepts each time, I continued reading them. The more I read, the better I understood the intensity of our psyche.

How The Subconscious Mind Affect Our Daily Life and Body

Our subconscious mind holds and controls everything in our lives. Practically every one of the things. It is certainly more than 95 percent; our entire lives have a place with our subconscious mind!

On the off chance that anybody tells you that there is no such thing as a subconscious mind, ask them back, "Would you say you are going to quit breathing, as your heart quits working? Does your blood course stop, does your food absorption stop while you rest? You are mindful of them while you rest?" They will say, no! At that point, solicit to them, what is controlling all of them.

I firmly suggest you read "The Power Of Subconscious Mind "by Dr. Joseph Murphy.

You will get a far-reaching general comprehension of it. Instructions on how to to utilize your intuitive mind to benefit from it and how to apply for better things throughout your life, etc.

How Subconscious Mind Makes A Habit

The main way we feed our subconscious mind is through our sensory faculties such as how we see, hear, smell, taste, and touch (this is technically our conscious mind). In spite of the fact that the subconscious mind is unarguably far more dominant than our conscious mind, it doesn't separate what is great or what is terrible.

Whatever we feed intentionally or unwittingly, our subconscious mind acknowledges it.

Sudden Hunch!

Let me reveal to you how I might discover this strategy to stop my nail-biting habit.

As I have been learning these things again and again, for as far back as three years, I was so curious of how I could apply these standards to practice to check whether these theories I have been perusing are a lie or not.

Bravo! Why can't I utilize these systems to stop my enduring habit throughout my entire life of biting my nails.

There are such a significant number of articles about nail-biting, YouTube recordings, web journals and so on! Be that as it may, they for the most part wind up promoting items like synthetic chemicals, soar oil, fake nails etc. I accept that some of them have few beneficial encounters, yet none of them approach somebody who is truly enduring at nail biting.

I need to share with you my strategy and be with you as an "ex nail-biter". I know the torment, the blame and enduring you have. On the off chance that there is another nail-biter in this world, who has chomped nails more than me, there ought to not be many. Trust me

These Are Not Remedies!

I need every one of my readers to ensure that these strategies I am clarifying, are unmistakably NOT remedies. It is a technique for understanding our habit a lot further to dispense with them. Like I have mentioned a couple of times in this book, cures are for the impacts. In any case here, we are setting off to the reason where it counts in the subconscious mind.

Here, you feed your subconscious mind what you need in the terms of how it can 'get' you. Ideas feeding your subconscious mind, which are completely opposite to the habit your carrying. When you educate your subconscious mind on the proper behavior, in the language it can comprehend, it will work for you and you will easily be able to accomplish anything your need in your life.

Without spending a penny to mystics, not addressing anybody/gatherings, not getting any help from anybody, you can get out from this habit as I did. At this point, I will promise you how it makes you stand with pride. How your public activities improve, (Nail-biting causing you feelings of inferiority), how certain you feel about yourself.

You realize the lovely part is, this is only the start. I can guarantee that you will feel total without the guilty emotions you were carrying for a considerable length of time, maybe even decades.

What Is Wrong With Therapies?

On the off chance that you are an obsessive nail-biter, I am certain you have attempted the vast majority of the things I have attempted up until now. Maybe it's more than I have attempted. I am certain you all have gone to treatment at any rate once in your life to get rid of this habit.

According to my observation, treatment could possibly work for you for one reason and one reason only! That reason is "REPETITION". Regardless of what sort of therapist, the method might be a Hypnotic specialist, Trans Therapist (that I attempted), or any other various techniques. If you don't take an interest enough for their sessions normally, your outcomes will finish up impermanent.

NOTE

You may stop your habit temporarily, but you may begin once more. This happened to me! I began my habit again after one year.

Why? The reason for me was that I had never taken part of routinely sessions as the therapist asked me to. Furthermore, this made new recommendations to my subconscious mind more fragile and my habit gradually started to rise.

The greatest obstruction for the vast majority of individuals is the investment, the heaps of cash you need to spend for every session. This includes the uncertainty you have that the cash you spend to them is commendable, you might begin the habit once more, or you don't have sufficient time or energy to go to them consistently because of your bustling life. The primary concern is, paying little mind to the technique you are using, all are working similarly!" They are conversing with your subconscious mind ".

That is it. All things considered, that is the thing that we are attempting to do here without paying anybody nothing. We are monotonously conversing with our subconscious mind in the language it comprehends, with attention to the habit we have.

What We Have To Do From Our Side?

This is critical to readers!

You purchased this book since you need to stop nail-biting, right? So here are the things you need to follow to get the best out of this book.

- Particularly take a strong, firm decision that you will overcome this habit by utilizing this book.
- You need a good understanding/awareness about your habit. Though you may find the initial chapters boring, and you don't come to the key aspect, I would recommend you read them often as they are important to feed our subconscious mind with this new model we are talking about here.

- You need more awareness with your hands and fingers.
- You need a little discipline and self control to do the activities day by day on many occasions, as explained in this book. These exercises are not hard at all. You don't even need a minute of your time once you get the idea of how to do these minor tasks. You will backfire all triggers coming to you to bite your nails within a matter of seconds.
- In the early stage, you need a small sacrifice to save a little time reading this book every day.
- Keep reading this book favorably in the chapter with affirmations.

NOTE

We live in a time buffer to manifest our dreams. Also explained in the movie "The Secret", this surely serves us. Otherwise, we could be in trouble if everything good and bad pops up in our life and we become overwhelmed by them.

This resembles that you don't need to worry about the time to get all the results you want. Just focus on the exercises and do them on a "repeated" basis.

CHAPTER FOUR

Sudden Hunch
(The law of vibration and the law of polarity)

The Law Of Vibration

As per Bob Proctor on his studies, we are living in an ocean of motion. Each and every thing vibrates. Everything integrates and disintegrates. As a molecular structure, each particle of our body is vibrating. The fascinating part is, our body vibrates as per our thought patterns. There are endless quantities of frequencies that are vibrating to a limitless number of thoughts we carry.

As you are most likely are aware, we as nail-biters' regularly chomp our nails while we are exhausted, strained, worried, irate, lonely and even hungry (that's me) and many other negative feelings I didn't refer to here.

So, are these feelings positive or negative? You know they are negative. These negative thoughts are making our body vibrate in a recurrence (bad Vibes), in a negative frequency which draws in negative things throughout our life. So, how we can apply this in our life?

Ask Someone How They Feel!

They would state "I am feeling magnificent, feeling awesome!". Or on the other hand, not all that well. "The previous couple of days truly dreadful".

NOTE

This implies they are clarifying their conscious awareness of the vibration they are in and the body.

So, presently, if somebody asks you how you are feeling while you are biting your nails, what might your answer be? Aren't you showing your feelings through biting your nails? Consider it.

Consider an obsessive nail-biter?

We should not be kidding here. The more we are into nail-biting, the more regularly we convey negative feelings with us, correct? This isn't great people. This isn't.

How To Fight Your Habit With The Law Of Polarity

The law of polarity exists from the beginning of everything. You know the law of gravity. Previously we have discussed the law of vibration and gravity. Just like that the law of polarity always exists.

What is the law of polarity? If you have to explain, "It is exactly the opposite of anything".

I got to know about this while watching a video of Bob Proctor. He mentioned this concept, everything has an exact opposite.

The most effective method to fight your habit is with "The Law Of Polarity".

You know the law of gravity. Already, we have talked about the law of vibration and gravity. Much the same as that, the law of polarity argumentatively exists.

How Can This Help Us? What Does It Tell Us?

I believe it suggests that we should constantly look at the good in people and situations, and that we should make a constant effort to slide up the pole of polarity. We know it is bad, but we should choose to look at the good, we should always choose to have good thoughts.

Why?

Good thoughts create good vibrations. Good vibrations attract good things.

There is always an opposite -- in a bad situation, you can "<u>CHOOSE</u>" what you want to concentrate on.

Have you ever thought that you had it bad? Then, something good happened and you were smiling for the rest of the day?

Have you ever thought that you didn't like someone, then someone else talks about how nice that person is, how well liked she or he is, how accomplished in an area that that person is? Have you ever hated the looks of a car, then someone you like bought that type of car and asked if you wanted a ride and you decided it wasn't such a bad car after all?

Why not consciously change your mind to see the good in everything? It's just too easy to slide down the pole of polarity into the negativity, isn't it?

Unless you choose not to, right? Then, it becomes a habit to slide up. The more you do it, the easier it becomes. Habits are done without much thought. You just do them.

Sudden Flash Of Polarity!

Imagine that you have an issue, I mean any issue in your life. There is an accurate inverse arrangement in your life. Truly, it is as straightforward as that. On the off chance that you are poor as indicated by the law of polarity, there is a careful inverse of it. Which means you are likewise rich.

If you are obvious about something, there is a precise inverse. You don't know about it, isn't that so?

In actuality, on the off chance that you have this awful habit for biting your nails. You got it, you are not biting your nails by any means.

If you have ugly nails and cuticles, what do you think? You have excellent, beautiful fingers and nails.

Dear readers, I can't express to you enough how significant this is. This flashed into my mind while I was watching Bob Proctor in a similar video a couple of times. I was supposing, how straightforward this all is? The dark-light, rich-poor, troubled-glad, where does this end? This is enormous! This is it...

Why we can't make a difference with this to our life. This is as basic as the law of gravity. Everything has an opposite. A bad situation is equally good. Look for the good, and more good will be on its way.

Or, how I like to put it, I can choose whether to label sitations good or bad. Looking for the good, will always bring peace.

A great way to practice the Law of Polarity is to start noticing the good things in your life. Part of the Law that I briefly mentioned is gratitude. Take 10 minutes at the beginning and the end of each day to think about the good things that have happened and express gratitude for them. Another thing I try to do is say a quiet thank you whenever I notice something good. Don't you like it when someone tells you, "Thank you!"? Doesn't it make you want to do more for that person? Same goes with the universe. The infinite power we all are under.

The New Model

What are the above illustrations? What is so special about this book?

We are building a new model to change the thought patterns we got so used to fueling the nail-biting habit. We are replacing the old thinking model. There is a nice word for that called "paradigms" to a new model. Fight the old paradigms or try to change them without replacing a new model is proved to be "totally worthless".

I need to present you with a wonderful quote which is one my favorite. Mr. Bob Proctor always mentions it in his teachings from *R. Buckminster Fuller*.

"You never change things by fighting the existing reality. To change something, build a new model that makes the existing model obsolete."

See how beautiful this is. How we can apply this quote to our life. This philosophy was explained in the movie 'Secret' as well. Imagine if you keep saying or thinking to yourself "No" to something or someone that you don't want or don't deserve, or something bad happens to you; our subconscious mind will attract them to you more and more as that is exactly the language you are asking it for. It will manifest to you.

Why?

Because of these encounters of things that you "DON'T WANT". There are many negative emotions such as anger, fear, envy, irritation, frustration, disgust that is dominating our minds. As I explained earlier, our body vibrates in frequencies according to the thought patterns and you guessed it, our body starts to vibrate in all these negative frequencies. So, what are you going to manifest in your life? Think about a person who carries all of these emotions always (maybe yourself). He or she also carries all of these bad vibes, always backfiring and disrupting throughout their lives.

The sad thing is, that they are blaming others for their own mistakes. This is sad but true.

Back to our nail-biting, for this habit here, we are building a new model to change our old "paradigms" with a new one through "AWARENESS" and "REPETITION".

The new model we explain here is going to replace nail-biting "paradigms", with a person who has new "paradigms" that as they don't bite their nails ".

CHAPTER FIVE

The Ultimate Decision & Sixth Sense

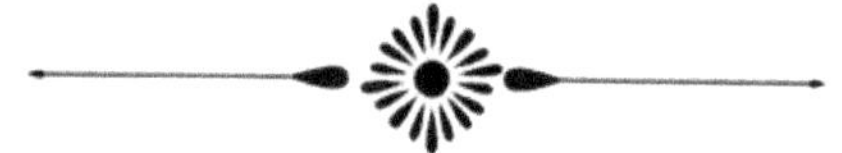

I'm sure, as of now, you are so desperate and are perhaps feeling impatient in coming to the heart of the matter, and you may be thinking, "When will this end? Let's get to business!". Well, sorry, but there is one more thing, probably the most important thing, for you to understand before we begin the process.

This little chapter will be a very short one but, nonetheless, the most important one. And for your record, I have added this chapter later and thought to put it before the beginning of the "Plan Of Attack" chapter, so it would be a nice kick start for you.

The Power Of Making A Decision

Starting with an unwavering decision to overcome nail biting, will make your mind stronger and ready for the process. Here, we are going to prepare a strong statement to say on a repeated basis to ourselves, until that idea soaks to the bare bones of our inner being (inner self).

So, how do you make that happen? You need to talk to yourself with feeling, you need to mean it! I promise you, even before we start, you will already feel amazing just after saying this to yourself.

There is another section in the next chapter about the same thing, but I have made the following more recently; which I believe it is more powerful than the one you are going to read in the post chapter. Also, as you will find out throughout my book, repetition is key; so there is no harm in doing it all again.

I'd like to put it this way, with a metaphor; assuming that you don't have a place of your own to stay, perhaps either staying with your parents or in a rented apartment. You have to think that it's time to move on, and it's time to buy a home rather than paying month-by-month rent. Staying put would not be a good idea at all! Your family is probably growing, and you're dreaming of buying your own "nest" to make sure that your little one comes into this world and has their own sweet home!

Now you want it so bad, keep thinking about it. Start your google search for a beautiful home. Look at those photos that match the home in your mind. At this current moment, you are wishing for a home for your family.

Then, here goes the big important question.

Have you decided to buy a home yet?

You see, this question is all that matters. Would anything happen until you decide to buy your dream home? It's a simple, yet powerful choice that you need to make! What is that question again?

> "HAVE YOU DECIDED TO BUY THE HOUSE OR NOT?"

You can day dream about it, search for images about it, talk to your friends about what you are planning, go to all of the places that you want. But have you DECIDED to buy the home yet?

YOU DON'T NEED TO SPEND A PENNY TO "DECIDE" TO BUY A HOME! RIGHT?

What do you think? Would anything under the sun really matter, if you still haven't decided on buying your dream home?

If you have yet to make that decision, then it's time to think like this...

"I will have my own home by next year in January, and I will move there with my partner, and we are going to have the baby in our own new home"

Just like that, it's crystal clear. Flat straight! You have DECIDED what you want. Clear?

It may feel awkward, and even thinking on deciding about your new home with your current set of information could be hard.

But what happens here is that your mindset (your thought vibrations) will move from hoping to buy, to "how to" buy the home.

You will start to think about how to find the money for your home and you will start to look for the home that you are dreaming about; perhaps even begin to contact real estate agents to discuss your options, and even go to the bank to talk to the manager about your financial requirements. As you can see, one thing starts the trend and leads to other events that bring you closer to your end goal.

Sooner or later, as we discussed in later chapters, your vibrations will work with the law of attraction and will bring you people and opportunities to make your dream home come true. This is science. It MUST manifest physically if you do it right and stay consistent with your goal. There is no doubt about it.

Let's go back to what YOU want from this book. You want to STOP nail-biting for sure. That's why you are reading this!

Then, here we are going to make a firm decision to stop nail biting. And I am going to give you a powerful sentence to repeat to yourself about the decision you are going to make.

"FROM THIS DAY FORWARD, I WILL PROMISE TO MYSELF AND FIRMLY DECIDE, THAT I WILL STOP BITING MY NAILS FOREVER. ALL OF THE SUFFERING, PAIN AND NEGATIVE FEELINGS THAT I CARRY WITH MYSELF WILL BE VANISHED!"

I WILL GET ALL THE HELP I NEED THROUGH AWARENESS AND KNOWLEDGE, BY GOING THROUGH THIS BOOK AND APPLYING THE TECHNIQUES EXPLAINED, UNTIL I STOP BITING MY NAILS FOREVER. THERE IS NO ONE OR ANYTHING UNDER THE SUN THAT IS GOING TO CHANGE OR STOP WHAT I HAVE DECIDED. I WON'T STOP UNTIL I OVERCOME THIS HABIT."

How do you feel when you repeat the above sentence several times? Repeat it again, again and again! Day and night. Write this down somewhere, type it in to your phone's notepad. Read it several times a day, and I promise you that you will feel like superman!

Napoleon Hill wrote "Decision", the longest chapter in his "Think And Grow Rich" book, because he understood how vital a decision is! He illustrated that some people have sacrificed their lives for their courage of Decision, which they will be remembered for at all times! Here is few examples that I have taken from his book.

- *Lincoln's famous 'Proclamation of Emancipation' was to give freedom to colored people of all America, and it cost him thousands of friends and turned his political supporters against him! Despite his assassination, which he expected, he showed extreme courage, and he made that decision for the good! He is remembered at all times!*

- *Socrates had made a decision to drink Hemlock (poison) rather than go against his beliefs. He showed incredible courage and hoped his death would serve as a lesson in believing in yourself, as he valued truth more than anything and stood by his decision.*

- *Napoleon's favorite, and in his opinion, the greatest decision of all times, was how fifty eight men signed their names on The Declaration of Independence in 1776, bringing freedom to all Americans. This decision could have resulted in had each and every one of them hanging from a gallows!*

Source: 'Think And Grow Rich' by Napoleon Hill

Here, you don't need to be remembered, or get hanged by making a decision. All you need to do is make a firm decision, that is all, simple. In this scenario, the worst would happen is you could've failed in decision making and go back to your nail-biting. But I am sure you don't want to go there!

> "SUCCESSFUL PEOPLE
> MAKE DECISIONS QUICKLY AND
> THEY RARELY CHANGE THEM OR
> CHANGE THEM AT ALL""
> UNSUCCESSFUL PEOPLE RARELY
> MAKE DECISIONS BUT THEY
> CHANGE THEM SO QUICKLY"

So which person do you want to be?

If you want to be successful in overcoming nail-biting, you must make a decision fast, and you should never change your decision, even if the world turns upside down!

The Image Concept

What I am going to tell you now, you may have never heard of; or if you have heard about it, I'm sure you've never given it a second thought.

Every thought that comes to our mind is associated with an image.

This may cause a controversy in your mind, because without realizing, that associated images came to your mind, even while you were thinking about this dubious fact? Did you notice that? It is nearly impossible, to think about anything without an image coming in to your mind. Your mind creates images that are associated with its thoughts. And these images are unique to you, you invented and presented them to yourself within a split second! Got the idea?

In one of the upcoming chapters, I have mentioned _the most lethal weapon_ that I had to use to self-defeat nail-biting, it was to think and imagine beautiful fingers and nails on my hands, when I had an urge to bite my nails.

Image concept is very important to understand if you think about how the mind functions.

The Ultimate Decision & The Sixth Sense.

If you are uncomfortable with the words "Sixth Sense", don't beat yourself up! There is absolutely no need for that. I took this from Napoleon Hill's "Think And Grow Rich" book, from the last chapter. He dedicated this chapter to someone who had followed thoroughly through all previous chapters in his book, only then could the reader try to understand this "Sixth Sense". Otherwise, this "Sixth Sense" would make "no sense" to anyone.

So, why have I alluded suddenly to the "Sixth Sense"? I just needed to give you a reason to read this marvelous "Think And Grow Rich" book, to learn the principles explained and understand how important they are!

Now, I don't need you to go and buy Napoleon Hill's book and start to read about the sixth sense, but to give you an idea what I mean by the "Sixth Sense " here is a quote from the book.

_"Make your subconscious mind work
with creative imagination"_

That's it. If you want to learn more, why not read that marvelous book of *Napoleon Hill* yourself. But it is your decision.

Let's see, how "to make your subconscious mind work with creative imagination". First, we need to use our imaginative power to make a scenario favorable to us, where you make that committed decision about stop-biting-nails once and for all!

NOTE

This exercise is optional, if you are not sure on what you are about to try, then you do not have to. But I see no harm in trying, as I did it too after reading this chapter. This choice is totally yours.

An Imaginary Council To Reveal Your Decision

Every night before you retire, close your eyes. Make sure there are no distractions or sounds, and imagine a meeting table. (A council table if you like).You look around and you can see your whole family sitting in the chairs, filling the room. You can imagine a nice big table with comfortable chairs all around, and your whole family smiling at you; parents, your other half, your children, your best friends, anyone who you are fond of. Remember, in this imaginary council, you are the president. You dominate this council and host it. Even your little baby, with the cute smile and good behavior, looks at you very attentively.

They all are so happy to give you their full attention! Imagine their faces with welcoming looks and smiles, excited to hear what you are about to say.

So here is what you are going to tell them:

"To all those who I hold dear,

For so long with so much pain, I have been biting my nails, and holding all of these negative feelings that have proved to be a great burden to me, and I have carried them with me. So, I have made up my mind, that I'm going to do something about it. From this moment today, I have stopped my nail-biting habit forever! I just want to let you know of this delightful news and I am now committed to make it happen!"

It's as simple as that, nothing else needs to be said. Then I need you to imagine that this exciting news makes everyone there look and feel incredibly pleased with your decision, each and every one of them congratulate you with cheers and clapping! I would recommend that you do this exercise mentally every day, as described, and you will find that as you practice this imaginary meeting, it will become more tangible. In the end, it will give you more and more courage to defeat your nail-biting habit. All of the scenes that you create in your mind, are more and more detailed and easy to make up. So that's your ultimate decision with a volunteered dream. To stop nail-biting forever, is your dream, right? Well, if not, then make yourself a dream,

> IF YOU DON'T HAVE A CLEAR DREAM, HOW CAN YOU MAKE YOUR DREAM COME TRUE?

CHAPTER SIX

Plan Of Attack

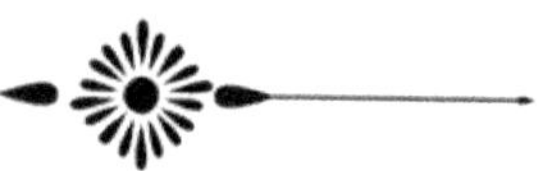

NOTE

This book, by far, clearly focuses on the habit of nail Biting. Remember, I won't promise, but you might try to discard other similar behaviors also with these comparable methods. But be assured, and I promise you that this is the path to beating your long-lasting nail-biting habit. If you have read the previous pages, you can understand why I have just said this.

Here, let us get back to our business.

> WHY PRODUCTS ARE NOT GOING TO HELP YOU? INDEED, EVEN IT MAY ADD MORE TROUBLES.

I am against every one of the items there are in the market to stop nail-biting, similar to phony nails, sour oils or different synthetic liquids. Whatever is on the market that I didn't specify, trust me, these are treating the effect, not the cause.

Why is focusing on the cause is so important?

THE CAUSE IS WHERE THIS HABIT RESIDES DEEP DOWN IN YOUR SUBCONSCIOUS MIND!

We have to deal with the cause, not the effect. To do so, we have to fix our subconscious mind.

It needs to hear us out and seize the habit. The key challenge here is how to cope with this habit in our subconscious minds.

As I have described before, individuals who speak about the nail biting habit and its psyche in my readings, eventually (a large portion of them) suggest for you to buy different items on the market because they have signed up to sell them for a commission. I am not against them, but they will not be of any benefit to us! One more thing about the goods on the market, is that we don't know what these chemicals are made of; I don't believe in them or how much damage they might do.

There are a few really important things you need to comprehend before we launch our plan of attack.

Be Aware Of Your Habit

It doesn't matter what therapy you've been going through in the past, one of the main reasons why you still haven't been able to quit your nail biting is that you have a tiny awareness of your habit.

You need to make sure that your subconscious mind knows what you're trying to get rid of, and not least, note that you need to make sure that 100% of the subconscious mind is on your side.

Rubber Bands,

Strap it on to your wrist, and every time you have an urge or every time you put your finger in your mouth, snap it to yourself. Really?

You are simply harming yourself. Forget it. I know, I tried it, it didn't work at all.

Fake Nails,

We are not used to nails. We are nail biters, correct? Truly! I'm still not used to nails. It resembles a blade that you dependably keep with you which you have no clue how to deal with it. Don't believe me? You should try washing your face with fake nails! You should try to clean-up or have a shower? What could they do to your eyes? Your skin is so delicate around your eyes and on the face.

Before we start our plan of attack, there are a couple of important things you need to understand.

Be Mindful Of Your Habit (The Awareness Level Of Your Habit)

If they want to bite their nails, I'm not saying a non-nail-biter would have more awareness, but when it comes to a typical nail-biter, we definitely aren't conscious of it.

There is not enough information or knowledge in our subconscious mind to be "aware" that we are chewing our nails and realize that it is not a good thing to do.

That's tragic! To improve the mindfulness of this habit, we should initially read a fair amount about nail-biting books (and also about OCD, Obsessive Compulsory Disorders) and take a look at what we are truly doing. I firmly prescribe you Google, and read a few articles about nail-biting, perhaps read a tad before you begin reading this book. Since it's important to understand at least the basic physiology about the habit of nail-biting.

Despite the treatment you may of had before, one of the most compelling motivations on why you couldn't stop your nail-biting, was that you paid minor attention to your habit. You have to ensure your subconscious mind comprehends what you are attempting to dispose of. Not least, again recall you have to ensure the subconscious mind is in your side one hundred percent to fight.

NOTE :

As I should be the first one who used this method, the challenging part is not to stop biting nails initially. You will obviously stop biting your nails once you have finished reading this chapter and understand exactly what I have explained here. It is the control and the elimination of the triggers and urges for nail-biting and maintain your mindset aftermath to the point where your subconscious mind flushes this habit once and for all.

Attack Now!!

Take A Committed Decision

Sit back for 15 minutes in your spare time, and think about a decision or choice you have made for your life recently. Have you made one or on the other hand <u>NOT</u>? On the off chance that you have made one, did you work hard for it? Building your dream home, or buying a home you love, or maybe you purchased your fancy sports car? Did that choice take you where you were trying to go? Or then again, did that choice cause you to have accomplished something in your life? If not, why?

Consider your life, does it suck? This is the casual term for all miseries we face in our life. I addressed myself a couple of years back, my life was truly exhausting.

Despite the comfortable and luxury lifestyle I have in Qatar, it was not fulfilled. But now I have transformed it in to something fascinating. Actually, all these because of how we think.

I would like to think about why our life is dreadful once in a while or more often, we don't have a settled target for ourselves to accomplish an objective. We may never have settled on a committed decision or a choice, and worked upon it until we accomplish what we need. If you approach somebody who is working hard for something better for their lives, the individual in question would answer "it's magnificent!". I have this arrangement, that they may not tell you what their plans are but they would never say their life is exhausting or sucks.

Think about this. Have you ever made a committed decision to stop your nail-biting habit?

What I meant with "committed decision", was a decision you made, that you are going to overcome this habit, nothing else!

Answer the following question...

Have you ever tried to use a method to overcome nail-biting? Though it might never work out, join a bunch of nail-biters for some group therapy sessions/meetings? Have you visited an online forum about this habit?

Anything at all? If you have not, whose fault is it? What are you going to accomplish if you've never tried anything?

My point here is that, before speaking to anyone, you need to talk to yourself first to resolve this habit.

With your soul and heart. This is how you talk to your deepe r mind, your subconscious mind!

I don't recommend that you join any groups, online forums or any other source where you have to address the same to pic over and over again. Think about it...

The more you do so, the more the habit wins, and that's wh at your subconscious mind feeds on.

Much like us, the same poor individuals are wallowing over stuff that you already know and experience "WILL NOT" hel p with anything at all. In reality, if you are involved with the m emotionally, it might fuel the habit.

Set The Goal For The Attack!

It is important not to feel bitter or ashamed about yourself if you haven't made a decision already, DO NOT! Here we are going to make one big committed decision, setting up a goal.

Here is the thing, go to a quiet calm place, probably your bedroom, sit back and relax, calm yourself and I need you to read following firm affirmation to yourself

"I will make a decision now to myself that from today, I will stop biting my nails once and for the rest of my life. I will have beautiful and healthy fingers on my hands after one year just, like any other." How do you feel after you said it to yourself?

The Law Of Polarity

Apply The Law Of Polarity To Your Nail Biting Habit

Now, we will see how we could apply the law of polarity to our nasty habit. I think this is the most important part of this whole book. I will try to put this simple as I can.

I have a little exercise for you, this is a "ONE-TIME" exercise to understand and be aware of our habit.

I need you to take an A4 piece of paper; draw a line in the middle of the paper, on the top of the middle line, write down "My nail-biting habit". In the left column, write down in bullet form, about your nail-biting habit. How you feel, what are the problems you are facing. I mean anything and everything you have to say about this habit. This is clearly defining your problem and the answer is going to be on the right side. Feel free, take your time, a nice quiet room without any distraction will give you a clear mind to put all these things together.

> WORRIED ABOUT PAPER SPACE
> RUNNING OUT? GET ANOTHER
> PIECE OF PAPER!!

NOTE :

If you are thinking about preparing this in a word processor, I don't say you shouldn't, but I believe it will give you more push if you write it down nicely.

Once you finish putting all together on the left side, for each bullet point, use the law of polarity. Write down the exact opposite sentence which makes the left bullet point void.

NOTE

Please would you do this exercise before reading further? I know you may not feel like it but, it is vital. So, chop-chop...

This is the most important step you need to take, and now I believe you already have your list. This list is strictly personal only to you and you only, and be very honest about it. It is important to make sure that you feel free to write all you have about this habit.

I will give an example to make it easier for you, some of whi ch are from my personal chart for you to have a better unde rstanding. I will open my heart to the good of you here.

I am a chronic nail-biter.	I will never bite my nails.
All my nails are crooked because of nail-biting	My nails and fingers are beautiful.
All my cuticles are damaged because of long term nail-biting.	I have beautiful nails.
I always bite my nails when I am stressed.	I am always relaxed without biting my nails
I feel so bad each time I bite my nails and cuticles off.	I am totally relaxed and feeling wonderful.
I feel guilty and inferior when I look at my fingers and nails.	I am proud of myself and always confident.
I feel inferior when I look at other people's beautiful nails and fingers.	I respect myself and others. Others respect me in return.
I do not feel confident when I am in an interview or when I am in a meeting.	I am always feeling free, happy and confident.
I always feel that someone is watching my nails and judges me.	I never feel bad or have any doubts about my fingers or nails as I no longer bite my nails.

My First Step.

What's our target here? We ought to stop chewing nails forever, huh? First of all, what we did here was set a goal, and it was clearly defined on a piece of paper. Research has shown that, if we write down a goal, the goal is more likely to be reached instead of just keeping the goal in mind. I trust that, period! For me, it was like night and day. Trust me, you have to write it down!

Why?

If we write something down, it is there. Flat Straight! You can see it, read it, and it is solid. If we keep a goal in our mind only, our mind would not be busy only to keep that goal, but also about other things. Other thoughts, in our daily life battle. So, it is highly likely our goals are swayed away and influenced by our thoughts. No matter how hard you try.

The writing part is over. Now keep that piece of paper with you in your table drawer and I will advise that you have to read only the right pane (Right pane and right pane only!) from time to time to freshen up these positive thoughts. The more often you read them, the better.

Forget about the left pane!

Never read the left pane. YOU DON'T do that! Cover it... tear it off! Do anything to get rid of it! You won't need to read it again.

You don't need to read something you don't want, right?

2nd Step

Using affirmations.

Why Are We Biting Our Nails?

It's a habit programmed in our subconscious mind. This started with a habit (search and read some articles about how we start a nail-biting habit), and with repetition and emotions, we have programmed it deeply in to our subconscious mind. We did this unconsciously.

So, this habit occurred by repetition, and must be eliminated with repetition, right?

This is the part where you are speaking to your subconscious mind. The best way to speak to your subconscious mind is through affirmations on repetition. This is the practical part we need to do.

So, I have made these affirmations for myself.
- I have beautiful and healthy fingers and nails.
- I am relaxed, my hands and fingers are relaxed.
- I am relaxed, I am fully aware of my whole body.
- I am now aware of my nail-biting habit, I am free from it forever.
- I am relaxed and free from all triggers of biting my nails.
- I make sure my nails are clipped rather than biting them.

NOTE

How to use these affirmations.

These are the affirmations I made for myself. You may use these or make by your own, it doesn't matter, also you can look for affirmations in such websites like **www.freeaffirmations.org**

Remember,

- To write all the affirmations in the present tense.
- To feel and believe yourself that you have already had it in your possession.
- To feel and believe that you are the person who has already overcome this habit. Try to feel them emotionally.

NOTE:

I cannot stress enough how important it is to visualize your gorgeous looking fingers and to feel for yourself that "They are your hands now". Just close your eyes for one moment, feel and believe that you have those magnificent fingers and nails. Just use your imagination, looking at your fingers side by side, and enjoy that now you have these wonderful fingers. You need to feel and believe yourself, that those fingers are your hands.

What is crucial is that you need to find the right statements that suit you. I am not going to argue over affirmations with you. You will certainly get an idea of what you want habit you want to get rid of. Feel free to use statements I've used, or any other statements to go along with your nail-biting exercise; just make sure you keep the list of statements less than ten because what matters is, getting your list of statements written or printed down. There is also another method, which is discussed in the following paragraph.

Use Your Smart Phone Instead (This is what I did most of the time)

If you are working in an office or if you are a busy person traveling, you can't keep a piece of paper on you that you can read all the time, so what I would suggest is that you grab your phone and have a notepad app installed to your phone (I used this) and type all of the affirmations in it.

Whenever you feel you need to bite your nails, just go through them once or twice. This way, people will never notice you are reading a piece of paper about "any end of the world prophecy," or think that you are losing it. Folks, you don't need that attention. Trust me, use technology!

When Do You Have To Read It? How Many Times?

For this question, my answer for when is, definitely in the evening, before you go to sleep and the first thing the morning. According to my own experience, I did it before I went to sleep. The more times that you read it, the faster your subconscious mind grasps your suggestion.

So, read as many times as you can per day!

Me, I read it less than 10 times, even in the beginning stage as a very heavy nail biter. (It takes less than one minute). You can read this while you are having a cup of tea in the office or during your lunch break. Actually, you don't need to disturb your normal life for this at all.

Use Imagination, visualize while you read affirmations.

I will explain to you what you will experience in this initial stage in the next chapter, but before the end of this, I need you to remember another important step.

You need to read as you mean it, these affirmations. Don't p ush it. The more affirmations you read, the more practice y ou get. I highly recommend that in the first few days, you re ad these affirmations as much as you can. But if you're in th e midst of another job and if there's any desire when you're tired, read-only once. That is enough.

Do not push this. In this method, there are no shortcuts. Co ntinuing the exercise is the most important thing. This is all that I did at the start and I will explain the stages I have passed in the next chapters.

NOTE

If you follow the above that I have mentioned step by step in the plan of attack chapter, I will personally guarantee that you will already have started to feel and believe that you have stopped nail-biting and I promise you will know it from the first day.

NOTE

Remember, you are in a silent war with your subconscious mind. If you force it, if you try to command it, you are one who is going to lose. Always remember to be friendly and in harmony with your subconscious mind. Be subtle with it. You don't want to mess with your boss alright?

A Nail-biting habit can be very irritating. It needs to be dealt with at grass-root level. One needs to overcome the psychological problems that are causing it. One can adopt simple measures to get rid of the habit. Sincere efforts need to be made to do away with the habit.

CHAPTER SEVEN

The Initial Stage

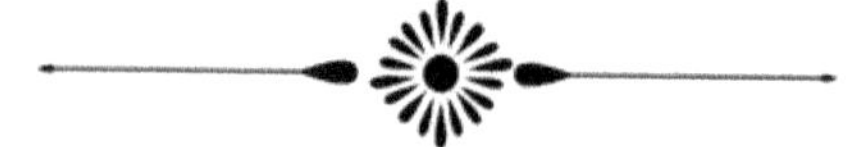

Time Of Excitement

Greetings! As I have explained, you have just started achieving something for your life. I had this excitement, the happiness, the feeling of fulfillment as now you are almost a "NONE" nail- biter.

Keep in mind to have a little discipline and commitment about the affirmations, and probably after one week, you will start to see the sunshine of your nails as they being to grow like a baby.

This excitement, the new energy made me avoid biting my nails in the beginning, almost completely. That doesn't mean you are done. The hard part was coming. Guess what? For me, I didn't even see it coming!

I will explain this to you in the next chapter.

You must have the discipline and at least a tiny commitment to read your affirmations daily as much as you can. If you prefer, I would recommend you using the same audiobook to also listen to while you drive or while you're at the gym, even use headphones at work if possible.

The more you feed these ideas, the more awareness you get to fight the habit, MORE QUICKLY WILL YOU GET THE CORRECT MINDSET!

For me, I've never forgotten to read it before going to sleep. How hard it can be to grab your phone and read the affirmations in it? I hope you can do it too! This is the best time to read your affirmations one by one as you mean it.

If you are a college student, it's easy. You are not married with children (I guess), so it should be super easy for you.

When you read affirmations, you can't have any distractions . It's not a big deal, as it will just take about ninety seconds to do this. As you mean, take all the time you want to read them. Have it your own way, but be dedicated and preserve your endurance.

Picture A Hand With Beautiful Fingers And Nails

From all the time we spent with this habit daily (this is repetition), we see out busted cuticles and nails and begin to get involved emotionally; we are feeding our subconscious mind about this habit that we don't want.

Note
Our subconscious mind doesn't know the good and the bad or understand them. The subconscious mind embraces and stores information whenever you think, say, or do something repetitively. This is a big issue we have to tackle.

> *"WHATEVER WE PLANT IN OUR SUBCONSCIOUS MIND AND NOURISH WITH REPETITION AND EMOTION, WILL ONE DAY BECOME REALITY."*
>
> *"EARL NIGHTINGALE"*

That is where I thought of a photo of a beautiful hand and nails. When you say the affirmation, "I have beautiful healthy nails and fingers", what is the first picture that comes to your mind? Your destroyed nails and cuticles? Then there is a problem we have to take care of.

That's why this picture is important. With this affirmation, feel and believe and visualize that you have those beautiful hands and nails at the moment. To do this, make sure to have a good memory of that picture. Google the photo. Make sure it suits your skin color. Take a printout of it. You will find thousands of them.

This is how you trick your subconscious mind! Be subtle!

In the meantime, I will also strongly suggest that you make t his picture available in a position where you will always look at it. Your office table, study table, perhaps, an open space where you walk by at home, just make sure you see it every time.

You can do this by finding an image on the Internet and prin
ting it out. Yet affirmations have more meaning. Only don't
do it if you can't keep a photo of this picture in your office.

What About This Habit For Children?

I am not a psychiatrist, who is teaching you any psychology
here. I am sharing this idea with you with my own experience
with NO side effects by any mean. But one thing for sure is, I
have had this habit since I was at least 5 years old.

I'm 36 years old now, and I have no idea what the psychics of
a child are. But as their habits are not as seasoned as adults,
I know it's easy to break a child's habit. I don't know if this is
going to work for a child, and I think this book should work
perfectly if someone is old enough to learn and understand
anything. I mean, look, for more than 30 years, I've been a
nail biter. To break this habit, I have done everything.

This is the only one that's been working for me.

CHAPTER EIGHT

The importance of Repetition

How to influence ideas to your subconscious mind (Paradigms).

Your subconscious mind is your most loyal, endlessly loving, friend in your life. It's your lifesaver and a best friend of yours. And when you are asleep, it takes care of you. It ensures that you absorb food, pump blood and all the essential functions of your breathing while you sleep, to keep you alive during your sleep. So, even when you are sleeping, the mind works 24/7.

Meaning, when you are unconscious. It makes no failures. It does what you say it to do, exactly.

One of the most significant aspects is that everything you saw, smelt, felt, heard and tasted is remembered. Each experience in your life remembered. It remembers not just everything, but everything in every little detail, every feeling we had, and so on and so on.

At least 95% of your whole being is taken care of by your subconscious mind. It is up to your deliberate choices, right or wrong. It is unaware of both its decisions and behaviors.

Paradigms

WHAT IS A PARADIGM? HOW BOB PROCTOR EXPLAINS IT?

Why do we have some habits that our parents do? Why do we have the same habits of other people around us? Have you ever thought about it? Why do we have the same or even more abilities than people who are rich and living their fuller life, but we are still broke and unhappy? We are sick, broke and just existing other than living the life we want?

The answer here is because of "Paradigms". We think, act and live our lives according to paradigms. We are "programmed". If you are waking up every morning at 7.00 AM, that is a paradigm. If you are always in debt, and the money you earn is not enough to enjoy your fuller life and maybe not even enough to pay your bills, that is a paradigm too. A paradigm is a mental program that operates in our subconscious mind (this programming happens unconsciously through our five senses) that controls and drives every encounter of our life. Paradigms are responsible for how we think, how we work, even how we sleep, etc. Whether these paradigms are good or bad, they all have been programmed by our environment we lived in and are living in currently. Paradigms are also accountable for our perceptions, as they are the way we think and judge and come to a conclusion about anything we encounter in our lives.

If you make fifty thousand dollars a year, Bob states, the paradigms are only set to make fifty thousand dollars a year. That means that you only know how to earn $50,000 a year.

If you are working in a company for more than twenty years, your paradigms make you happy living with what the pay check offers you.

Think about how many paradigms you deal with, and whether you want to change them. Now, you know that the book you're reading here is also about a Paradigm as well. That'd be nail-biting!

Although it does a lot of physical and even emotional damage to you, somehow recognized by our subconscious mind as part of our lives.

How Paradigms Influence Our Life?

You will also understand how paradigms have an enormous effect on your life, and no matter how much you try to change the circumstances of your life, if your paradigms do not change, nothing can happen.

Let's take a metaphor, as this habit (nail-biting) is profoundly rooted as a concrete building in our subconscious mind. Unbreakable, it seems. You must demolish it anyway. There's no one supporting it for you. How do you do that? You should first take one sledge hammer and, let's say we began using a sledgehammer and to hammer it down. How long would it take? How much effort has to made to completely demolish the building with the sledgehammer? You hit walls and concrete and, the more you hit the more matter that is going to separate from the building.

Consider this book of yours as the sledgehammer for you to break this habit. How you are going to use the sledgehammer as explained in the plan of attack?

Here we are REPEATEDLY hitting a nail-biting habit with affirmations, opposing it and slowly the building is going to collapse. We are PERSISTENTLY replacing the habit we have with a new model. If you are NOT using these techniques, persistently on a repeated basis, it would to be least effective.

If you are planning to follow instructions in this book timidly, tentatively; I would say you rather not read this book at all. Persistence and repetition is the key.

If anyone has a question about how persistent and repetitive you should be? Well, that usually depends on how big your habit is and how soon you want to get rid of the habit. More often as we can, we need to express opposite ideas against our habits and that is what this book is about.

You need to read this book more frequently as well! The subconscious mind sips these "New Ideas" Much easier if you can also get the audiobook to listen to it. When you drive to work and return home, you can listen to an audio book. Believe me, it helps a lot.

If you want to get rid of this habit sooner, then do exercises more often on a repeated basis.

Slowly, your subconscious mind flushes away your habit and plants new ideas opposite to your habit, and soon there will be no place in your mind for the nail-biting habit.

"The concrete building will become completely demolished"

The Only Way

<u>The only way to remove any habit, including the one we are talking about here (nail-biting), is to impress new ideas and thoughts against the habit repetitively.</u>

There are no remedies required for this. No products or any other individual needs to get involved with you in this process. You can find all those ideas (affirmations) and thoughts from this book itself. Keep planting new ideas through repetition until your paradigms, with old habits, completely replaces them with new ones. Then you will gradually start to act and behave according to new paradigms you have planted by yourself.

NOTE

I have learnt that there's another way of changing paradigms from Bob, which is a big emotional impact. A big emotional impact means that something wonderful or terrible happens in your life which affects you deeply and you involve yourself deeply and emotionally with it.

For example, an individual may become a totally strange person if he/she loses a loved one in their life. The persons existing paradigms shift because they are deeply being involved with sad and destructive feelings. That changes the paradigms. You might have seen individuals like that. Especially youngsters.

The subconscious mind doesn't know the difference between what is real and what is unreal.

Even if our subconscious mind remembers something, remember that we spoke about it, remember that it can't decide what is true and what we imagine. We are still accepted by our subconscious mind, whether imagined or actual, by thoughts and experiences. What is your habit of nail-biting? You know, it's no good. But with guilty feelings plus several other negative feelings, we have already begun and done it for so long. How will it go away, then? Got my point?

Take advantage of your subconscious mind, it accepts anything! It doesn't matter if it is real or not.

NOTE

If you feed an idea (any idea regardless) your subconscious mind accepts all of it, and if you feed the same idea on repetition (regularly), it sinks deep down to your subconscious mind. Once that idea sinks to your subconscious mind, it makes sure you act upon that idea. Then they attract and manifest in the future. (Bob Proctor)

It doesn't matter whether your idea is about getting sick or getting rich. It accepts and gives it back to you. Period!

The Conscious Mind Is The Filter

Our conscious mind is the main filter, having the ability to determine which ideas to be sent or not to our subconscious mind. That's why I have mentioned here many times, the importance of a positive mindset.

We need to try our best to stay in a positive mental attitude more often (on repetition), so that they will come to manifest in our lives. If we do so, we will start to reject negative emotions effortlessly.

Example (my personal encounter)

I used to watch war movies and horror movies that I was abl e to watch without any difficulties with audience discretion advice, blood and murder. But now I cannot comfortably wa tch them. I generally watch comedy movies more often.

Note, habits of thought rely on ideas coming from your subc onscious mind. The more we feed positive thoughts to our s ubconscious mind, the more it generates positive thoughts, ideas and feelings.

Repetition of positive affirmations that we desire, is highly effective. If you want to absorb any idea, literally any idea, the best way is to write down. You have it on a piece of paper and read it aloud to yourself. It is proven for best results. The best times to read these affirmations are just before you retire in the night and the first thing in the morning. Because at this time your mind is sentimental from other emotions and the more sentimental your mind is, it is easier to feed ideas to your subconscious mind.

Holding Positive Thoughts (Uninvited Visitors)

We sometimes have visitors to our home. Maybe your life partner came to your life as a visitor in the first place. Do you know that you get around 70,000 visitors to your mind per day? Who are these visitors?

These are known as thoughts. These visitors come to your mind, linger for a while, and move on, leaving space for oth er thoughts. Know
that our brain processes these thoughts and we are the only
 creatures that are completely disoriented with thoughts co ming into our brain. Since they are mixed with their world,

all other creatures act upon them immediately. As people, we have the capacity to accept or reject them. Rationalizing them, too. I love this idea.

Note

Think about this a little deeper, you will understand how significant this is. What are the advantages we have with our gifted mind over other animals? This is like a free menu, given to us to choose anything and everything we desire.

Dominating Thoughts

So, here, we need to realize what we've been doing in the p ast, whether we've been generating positive thoughts and p reventing negative thoughts or vice versa.

If you can process incoming thoughts as positively as you can, then those dominant thoughts can eventually sink into your subconscious mind (on repetition). If you let in negative feelings as well, the same thing happens. And what would be the difference between the dominant thoughts of these two kinds?

Your entire body vibrates according to the sort of dominant feelings you have, according to the law of vibration.

This means that the body vibrates at a similar frequency if you are always satisfied and optimistic.

And when your body vibrates at this frequency (happy vibes) according to the law of attraction, the universe will match that frequency and attract the same. And now you know wh at would happen if you wereworried, upset, irritated and so on with your dominant thoughts. Right?

NOTE

To learn more about this, I strongly recommend you watch some YouTube videos of Mr. Bob Proctor, read his book "You were born rich ". There is a whole chapter for the law of vibration and also read Dr. Joseph Murphy's "The power of the subconscious mind ". You will learn these in a whole lot of detail. Remember, nail-biting has already become our habit. So, how do we fight the habit?

"By constant repetition of thoughts which are the same opposite of your habits".

This is the only practical way of dominating your subconscious mind and shift habit patterns. Remember, your subconscious mind acts on what thoughts you are feeding it with daily. In this case, make your conscious mind the boss who filters only and particularly positive thoughts to your subconscious mind. You do this and see where your life directs you, and watch how magic starts to happen!

CHAPTER NINE

The Interim (THE Hardest STAGE)

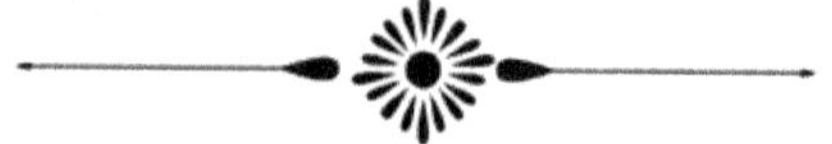

As discussed in the initial stage, you're halfway through this enthusiasm and energy and the rewarding feeling you will forever have. Since you may have stopped biting your nails entirely, there is a rough time ahead and this chapter is also the practical part of all the actions you have to take to conquer your unconscious mind. This is the key chapter for your goal.

We still need to dig deep and keep feeding polar opposite ideas to our subconscious mind. Remember? Demolishing the building?

Should We Worry About The Time?

Let Mother Nature grow your nails as she always does. Don't be so worried about how fast they grow.

Don't dwell on this particularly. Just go and take care your other businesses.

Also, don't worry about the time it takes you to completely stop the nail-biting habit, and the most important thing is...

"DON'T GET DISCOURAGED"

Keep on going and remember whenever you feel like biting your nails, visualize those beautiful fingers and nails. The time it takes depends on how you influence your subconscious mind and how much your subconscious mind is seasoned with this habit. The most important thing is to keep doing this small exercise continuously.

"PERSISTENCE & REPETITION"

Occasional Biting

Don't you worry about it! Don't feel bad or pity yourself. I also bit during my own process. Now I have completely stopped. That's why in my method, I never force myself (this is subconscious mind you are messing with). What we have to do is slowly feed positive ideas. Think about those beautiful fingers and nails of yours. The urge surely goes away.

What I can assure you is that from the moment you start this exercise, it will reduce at least 50 percent of your nail-biting. The rest is depending on how you understand and do the exercises frequently. When you start this process, you will realize within two weeks, that your nails start to grow, also the skin and cuticles around your nails.

You should be happy about this improvement and thank yourself about having succeeded to a certain level with this method. I fell in love with this method. Felt satisfied and happy about the progress.

I have managed to stop this within two months. Remember I was a chronic heavy nail biter. <u>I have NOW STOPPED THIS COMPLETELY.</u>

I never feel like I want to bite anymore, but instead, if I feel any nail or hanging skin, I would rather clip them.

MOST IMPORTANT!

NEVER WORRY ABOUT HOW YOUR NAILS, CUTICLES, AND SKIN GROW OVERTIME! THAT'S NOT YOUR JOB. YOUR BODY WILL TAKE CARE OF THAT BUSINESS. JUST KEEP DOING EXERCISES EXPLAINED IN THE BOOK. IF YOUR NAILS AND CUTICLES ARE DAMAGED BECAUSE OF PROLONGED NAIL BITING, IT TAKES TIME. A LOT OF IT! KEEP IN MIND, THE MOST IMPORTANT THING IS WHETHER YOU ARE BITING YOUR NAILS! NOTHING ELSE REALLY MATTERS!

"YOU MAY CLIP HANGNAILS INSTEAD TO KEEP YOUR URGES TO A MINIMUM"

I WOULD RECOMMEND THAT YOU HOLD THESE METHODS FOR YOURSELF ONLY, TO AVOID THE OPINIONS OF OTHERS THAT COULD HAVE AN ADVERSE IMPACT ON YOUR PURPOSE HERE.

THESE DAMAGED / BROKEN NAILS BELONG TO YOU. YOUR BUSINESS IS NOT WORRYING ABOUT THEM. PLEASE DO MIND YOUR OWN BUSINESS. I BELIEVE THAT IT WON'T HELP YOU IN THE PROCESS TO WALLOWING ABOUT WHAT YOU DO IN SOCIAL MEDIA. PLEASE DO YOURSELF A FAVOR... DON'T WALLOW LIKE A CHILD.

INSTEAD, WHY DON'T YOU CHALLENGE YOURSELF TO DO THESE EXERCISES? STOP NAIL-BITING COMPLETELY, AND FEEL FREE TO POST THOSE IMAGES ON YOUR FACEBOOK BEFORE AND AFTER A YEAR! HOW ABOUT THAT?

What To Do When You Are Feeling To Bite Your Nails?

Close your eyes, take a deep breath and say to yourself, "I have beautiful and healthy hands. And my hands and fingers are relaxed without me biting my nails".

"I am relaxed, my hands and fingers are relaxed without me biting my nails."

ONLY TAKES FEW SECONDS!

Remember your mind can give commands effective immediately. It's your mind that controls your whole body. Particularly your subconscious mind, as it takes part of that over ninety five percent! That's doesn't mean you can give commands consciously any less. Make the best of it!

Clipping (Important)

What I always saw was hanging nails, or small pieces of nails, or even raw skin which would touch my other fingers that led me to bite my nails. To be honest, when I feel a hang nail or skin, I always had a little look and nibble at my fingertips. Now, I'm working on it.

About causes, I can't say enough. We must battle with our t riggers in this point, so it will cease returnin. We must be ca utious. Remember, we should clip cuticles and any other hangnails. If you don't, your subconscious mind will remember it, and make you bite whether you like it or not! You probably don't even know about it consciously! That's for sure. I always clip it. Keep nails and use the clipper to shape extra skin.

"Don't Force It"

This is important. You can't force your subconscious mind to do anything consciously. There is a language that it listens to you. This is all about suggestion.

At this time, probably after one month after you started this exercise, and all the excitement and happy feelings are slowly fading away. And I can understand it. It is now sometimes when the old habit comes back to action.

Maybe you will realize this even after your finger is already in your mouth. Don't be disappointed, remember how long this habit was with you. Persistence is very important.

Note

Affirmation reading on a repeated basis is vital.

This might just be the first time that all these ideas (extra information) is bombarding against your subconscious mind. Suggestions should be given slowly and orderly to the subconscious mind. Subtle we have to be! Here, affirmations that we repeatedly read are essential in combating triggers. You could become frustrated if you push this too hard (which you were before)!

Remember? Take a deep breath with your eyes closed and think about those beautiful fingers and nalls. It always worked for me! It only took five seconds. There is no pressure here, nothing is hard. It will discretely deceive our urge and give more importance to what we want. Don't worry about how many times you tried it and how many times this trigger comes, once this method becomes a habit, triggers will come less often. Also, you can focus on more opposite thoughts. You can do this exercise every time the urge comes while you are busy at your office as well. Whenever you have time to settle down at the office for a few minutes, simply go through the list of affirmations in your mobile.

The Mind Trick Of Taking A Gander At Your Nails.

Presently, your subconscious mind truly misses biting your nails. It's now processing something new to deal with the habit you have been bringing through the years, or maybe decades like me. Let me clarify what my subconscious mind did when it missed biting nails.

At the last pace, while I was doing this exercise, I began to look at my nails more and more frequently.

This is important!

At a glance, I could see that my nails have developed; but why do I still look at them so often? To enjoy your improvement? Or you still need to bite them?

To be honest with you, I think my urge was deep in my mind and I felt as though I still needed to bite them. What did I do? Nothing. I just carried on the same exercise. (This is repetition.)

Note:

This is worth mentioning to you here. I particularly did the visualizing part whenever I had the urge to look at my nails. As soon as I wanted to look at my nails, I quickly distracted those thoughts with, "I have beautiful nails and fingers right there in my hands".

CHAPTER TEN

After Results (FINAL STAGE)

Do I Truly Feel Like Bite My Nails Any Longer?

Roughly after 2 months

My straight answer is NO! No more... I am completely done. I am so grateful, and I am so happy with myself about what I have accomplished. Following a few months (in less than three months), I see my nails are steadily growing and the most joyful part is, I clip them once in each three to four days. I think clipping my nails will additionally give more space and resources to develop cuticles. This is where I mostly lacked due to my nail-biting habit. I feel the tips of my fingers are getting increasingly rough. My fingernail skin is developing and forming as I always wanted.

Keep note to yourself:

Do not waste your time expecting your cuticles to grow faster than they are supposed to. It's a long process. Just be happy and proud about yourself. The most important things is, whether you are biting your nails anymore or NOT? Isn't it? If you are NOT, that's it!

Don't worry about the process of developing your cuticles which might take couple of years. Clip them once in a while. And happily go about your other businesses. I will update you in post scripts about my progress.

How Good They Are Now? (After Six Months.)

Still not perfect looking. I need them to be better. In any case, I do still clip them and I can observe my fingernail skin growing on a satisfactory scale. I enjoy my progress here and I'm taking pride in it.

Presently, I can open my mobile battery spread with my nails. I would now be able to open the plastic cover of the charging port of my Bluetooth gadget. I am never again feeling sensitive at my fingertips. No more infections! No inferior emotions! No blood! No pain!

Though still, my hands are not perfect, I have no feelings of hiding my hands away. That's the best thing I am feeling now.

No guilty feelings. I can hardly wait to see them develop fully and see how they look in the coming years.

I am so happy and grateful that I have conquered the habit of nail-biting once and for all.

Presently, I can concentrate on anything I need without biting my nails. If I get on the edge or whatever other triggers that previously activated me to bite my nails, I never put it all on the line. Maybe I may have been taking a tiny peek at my fingers unknowingly, so what the heck?

Just work on the same technique.

Despite all these, I do the little exercises often, this helps me to accomplish my nail-biting habit. However, for me very less often.

___My most valuable weapon___ *of all these techniques is simply picturing those delightful nails and fingers, feel and believe as they are right there in my hands.*

On the cosmetic perspective, this stage could be improved if you consider taking more vitamins to help your nail growth. I am not sure. I never used any. But if there is something proved to be helpful, why not? You've earned it at this stage!

I know and have heard of a few big celebrities who bite their nails, burn a large sum of dollars for phony nails and other different products. Does that solve this issue?

A resounding No! It doesn't. That is what I have been telling you all the time we should battle the reason. Not the result.

There is no point in putting a plaster on the wound when it's infected!

CHAPTER ELEVEN

Hypnosis vs this book

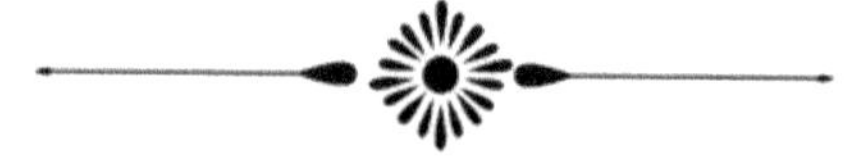

Since hypnoses has been a fascinating subject for me ever since I was a child, I thought to dedicate a small chapter in this book to my reader's reference, and for the record, hypnosis will also give a heads-up beating to the nail-biting. Here, readers should understand that I am not encouraging anyone to participate for any money burning hypnotic sessions to overcome nail-biting habit, but of course, I believe hypnosis should also work.

Hypnosis has been commonly understood and labeled by the normal public, used as a mere parlor trick method to charm people; or if you are even more paranoid "Do bad things", and more to stage shows and other performances, not an ideal psychology treatment method. It's a proven fact by scientists that hypnosis has very real and very positive effects in overcoming habits. Including nail-biting.

Hypnosis is NO placebo or any voodoo technique, and from the recent past, people have been realizing this fact. Hypnosis can be used for many things when it comes to psychic healing. You might have seen or even tried that there are a lot of MP3 audios that allow you to self-hypnotize yourself and talk to your subconscious mind and overcome challenges.

I, personally have never tried these mp3 audios, so I am not going to be the judge to say they are good or bad compared to a patient with a professional hypnotist.

NOTE

This information is for your knowledge only, that this doesn't resemble the need to go for any hypnotic sessions along with this book. All information about my methods and techniques explained in the book here, is enough for you to overcome the habit. But I need you to understand that "hypnosis" is not a "mind trick" which some people believe to be totally "fake". Every bit of it is as effective as say this book is.

Here are some pros of Hypnosis

- Hypnosis can cure phobias.
- Hypnosis would help a mother make herself relaxed and comfortable enough to give birth to a child in the most convenient way possible.
- Hypnosis can cure obsessive compulsory disorders (OCD's). That includes our "nail-biting habit".
- Hypnosis can cure addictions.
- Hypnosis can increase work/study performance.
- Hypnosis can increase your self-confidence/self-esteem.

- Hypnotic surgery while the patient being hypnotized contains absolutely no torment in the area they are being operated upon.

In the event that somebody looks for hypnotherapy to defeat any habit or any undesirable urgent conduct, they should get help from an expert hypnotherapist, which is costly. This book covers all that a hypnotherapist is commonly doing. The hypnotherapist would have different mesmerizing sessions with you and it relies upon the inducing subject of how often the number of sessions required. What's more, each time the patient must pay the charge and time requested by the trance inducer.

So, I emphasis the advantage of this book you are reading. Here we read the book on a repeated basis, comprehend its ideas, have great mindfulness and wipe out the nail-biting habit.

You can read this book at your own pace, time and accommodation.

So How Does It Function?

Rather than we have been practicing our exercise in the chapter "Plan Of Attack" to calm and relax and doing the visualizing technique on the repeated basis, in hypnotherapy when the subject is relaxed, he is in the "trans" state and open to acknowledging thoughts and recommendations on a subconscious level. In this state, his mind is spoken directly to his subconscious levels, new recommendations are being given to supplanting his "old paradigms".

"Repetitions are important with hypnosis too!"

These suggestions and new convictions must be fed on a repeated basis until the subconscious mind completely wipes out "current habits" and supplants it with new suggestions against it. Only a couple of sessions generally would prove to be effective, the patient could stop the habit for a brief period yet at the same time, they are taken back there until the "next" trigger springs up.

To eliminate, habits must be dealt in their subconscious level where a new automatic habit patterns are set up. That is what hypnosis sessions do to the subject. Habits, whether they are good or bad, are deeply rooted in the subconscious level of mind, which is beyond the senses for any human, as those habits exist as you do them even without noticing. But the human mind is always open to easily establish a new set of behaviors and habits as necessary, If we can feed them on a repeated basis until they slip into the subconscious mind. That is the magic and the beauty of it.

Habits are unconscious and to understand this, you would not wake up in the morning and say to yourself "Today, I am going to bite this much of my nails on my fingers and keep some for tomorrow". But as a matter of fact, you are exactly doing it, Right?

So, as long as habits are hidden beneath your conscious levels of mind, no matter how hard and how desperate they have to be stopped, you can't.

To start with, the hypnotherapist would discover what could be the driver or the explanation behind the habit, regardless of whether it could be a strain, dread, tension, etc.

The hypnotherapist will discover the underlying driver and he could play out a couple of basic broadly acknowledged schedules to treat the habit.

Affiliation

A hypnotherapist could connect the unwanted conduct to something really horrendous.

Model:

Recommending the subject, each time he attempts to bite his nails and when his fingertips arrive at the mouth, he will taste the inconceivably disturbing flavor.

Substitution:

Replacing the undesirable behavior with an increasingly attractive and innocuous one. Most individuals who chomp and/or chew their nails are embarrassed by the appearance of their hands/fingers and will hide their hands from sight. The reverse habit could be applied in the longing to have attractive nails/hands through good grooming habits.

Anchoring :

It would be the recommendation that sets up both affiliation and substitution in the subconscious mind. This could be that the subject is getting an awful taste or a smell each time they see their fingers going to their mouth and substituting each time, and the longing for appealing hands and fingernails.

Note

The root cause for nail-biting would be low self-esteem, which could also be replaced by suggesting new ideas of high self-esteem and confidence, allowing the subject to take pride in his self-image.

Stopping a terrible habit is easier when you are fully mindful of it. Each time you find yourself thinking of doing it, on the off chance that you know about it by sustaining thoughts against the habit to your subconscious mind, habits have no spot to vanquish in your brain.

Hypnotherapists likewise, could utilize neuro-linguistic programming methods (We are not going to talk about it in this book). This is a moderately new logical technique that will program the patient's brain to dismiss the inclination of any habits entirely. In conclusion, hypnosis for nail-biting has consistently had positive results in numerous individuals. The length of this method differs from one adviser to another.

CHAPTER TWELVE

Thank You Bob Proctor!!

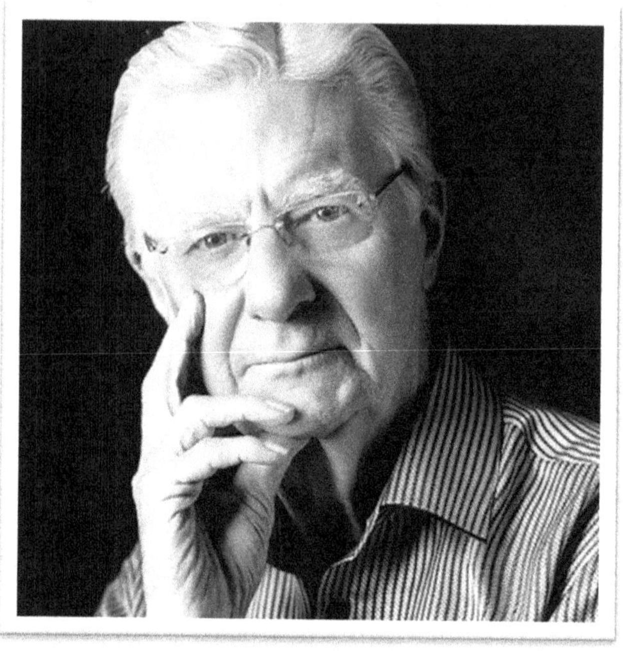

Image copied from Mr. Bob Proctor Official Twitter Account

"SET A goal to achieve something that is so big, so EXHILARATING THAT it excites you and scares you at the same TIME"

Bob Proctor

I was in a large dilemma about placing this chapter first or last. Then, I made a choice to put it last because I should not sway from the purpose of this book. Last but not least, I'm so grateful to this brilliant man, Bob Proctor, who altered my life. He became my mentor for the previous three years after watching "The Secret".

"What do you really want?"

That is the question where Bob captured all of my attention from the movie "Secret". I was so skeptical about what he asked there. No one has ever asked me that question in my whole life. What do I really want? First time I heard that from him, he got all my attention and I realized he is going to give me anything I need. What was the deal as to why he asked that? So, Let me watch the whole thing. (The Secret)

Well, yes, you were spot on their Bob!

I have been learning what he educates for, a decent lot starting from the fall of the year 2016 and as of now, I keep watching him, hearing him more often . Likewise, as he encourages, I regularly hear Napoleon Hill's 13 Success Principles in 30 minutes while I am heading to work each morning and night.

Being frank if I hadn't written this book, truly I would be a similar nail-biter as I was and last but not least, I would be the same person as I was with terrible circumstances and life, if I was not lucky enough to see Bob Proctor in the movie "The Secret" .

I wish one day, I could warmly greet this man and look in his eyes; and I might certainly wet my eyes with tears at that moment, because I am so grateful to him.

For sure one day, I will understand fully what the secret is. About the secret, Bob is telling others that anyone who wants to know "The Secret" should get that idea by themselves; meaning that they should by themselves, have a correct perception of what the secret is! And I may have a tiny glimpse of it by now, I keep studying it. I keep reading. The more I study, the more I understand the concepts and ideas behind the "Secret".

Dear readers, aside from us carrying this nail-biting habit, we are also carrying so many negative vibrations. Vibes of tension, doubt, frustration, fear, or perhaps even terrible depression.

Note

This isn't pinning out. Nail-biters are <u>NOT the only people</u> who carry these negative feelings.

However, I am almost certain none of us would nibble our nails off in the event that we are in an inspired state. To avoid that, we need a general understanding of these things.

You surely come to know these if you also study Napoleon Hill's 13 principles. I strongly recommend you all read Napoleon Hill's "Think and Grow Rich" book on a regular basis. That's how Bob Proctor started his wonderful life from "his misery". That's what Bob teaches us to get away from "our miseries". Awareness through knowledge is greatly an important thing we need to be close within our lives.

I have a suggestion for you. Watch the movie "The Secret". Watch Bob Proctor's videos. Watch other inspiring personal help videos. They all say wonderful things again and again. Sign up for those programs if you can.

If you still can't, there are loads of free information available on YouTube, and the internet. I would also recommend to you Bob Proctor's book "You were born rich", which he gives away in his website and costs you nothing. Just download it and read it. Read it more often.

When you read these remarkable books like Napoleon Hill's "Think And Grow Rich" more often, you will always live with the souls of those magnificent people like Andrew Carnegie, Napoleon Hill, Thomas Edison, Henry Ford, men we never met yet always remembered, who'll live everlastingly as long as the humankind exists. And bonus, countless "Aha" moments.

It will build you slowly to grow like them, work like them, think like them.

Say "yes" to your "Unconscious Competent". It's always looking for the perfect you!

Keep reading as many times as you can. Read each and every page again and again! There are years of information you could grasp in each chapter for sure!

Do me a favor in return, put your word about this book as a review for future improvements and deliver this message to people as much as you can.

Final Thought

I believe as you are reading this final chapter, you have already completely stopped your nail-biting habit or, at least are in the initial stage. All the chapters are from my personal encounters. Like I explained to you earlier, they are all honest and extremely personal emotions I had to go through with nail-biting which I had for more than three decades.

I wanted to open my heart and help you all to get rid of this through the method I used once and for all. Show confidence. Show your fingers while you are at the board meeting. Tell your bosses what you want to tell them. There is nothing to hide in the job interview.

No more worries about someone watching your hands. All these things while your fingers and nails are growing healthy and beautifully.

Keep this book as your companion at all times. At least for the first six months. Remember the affirmations exercise I explained to you when you feel like biting nails. I strongly suggest that you read at least one chapter from Chapter 5 before retiring at night. Also, remember affirmations on your mobile!

Also, remember to tell your friend, your sibling or anyone who you know or do not know who needs help! Once you're done, share this book with them. Make their fingers and nails beautiful too!

Keep reading books I have recommended to you. Read other books also. Read! It will change your life.

Period! A well-written book is a work of someone who may be with years or decades of research and study summarized in one place. The best example I know is Napoleon Hill's "Think And Grow Rich" There is nothing more better.

Know that I don't market anyone here. I am just telling you what I have done and what I am doing. I didn't sign up for any marketing campaign for anyone along with this book.

But I don't want anyone or anything not to be noticed in this book who helped me to write it knowingly or unknowingly and deserves a token of appreciation. That is the least I could do for those wonderful people!

Make sure you always feed positive ideas to your inner being at all times. It will listen to you, work day and night tirelessly to attract better things to your life.

Read this often. Don't give up. That is important. "Feed ideas against your habit of nail-biting." This is the cure I presented to you in this book.

Maybe we will meet again with another book. Do me a favor, just tell me what you have achieved from this book. Also, if you feel if this little book is worth reading and is helpful, be kind to put a good word on it as a review on the platform you read this. It will help future improvements and to deliver this message for all who are suffering from nail-biting!

Peace!

COULD YOU DO ME A FAVOR?

If you enjoyed this book, cherished, please put your honest thought about it as a review on the platform you bought it. It will help this book reach more people and also <u>future improvements</u>.

Asanka.

POST CHAPTERS

It's been almost 8 months since I have published this book and I thought that would be it with all chapters. But of course, it's NOT! As I have already passed my message about how to overcome nail biting using "methods" I used, it's not enough to just sit back and wait until people get my message further. While I am sincerely grateful for all the readers who spent their time reading and believing in this book, I thought of adding a bonus with "post chapters" with information about encounters that I was dealing with in people seeking a nail-biting solution. So please expect new updates consistently. If you have already bought the book, please write to me on my personal email address, I am more than happy to send you the newsletter pdf with new inputs.

I never forget my fellow readers who already trusted and spent their time to read my book.

EMAIL: ASANKAJAYARATHNE@HOTMAIL.COM

Note: I just made a blog! You need to check that out!

HTTPS://RICHMINDSECRETS.COM/

You can check this out now as I have included some contents further in my book and actually it's made as a landing page. This will surely will have some video lessons with my Nail-biting support group. This email will be always available, but I will keep you posted for any future email addresses comes up.

These "Post chapters" are not lengthy but interactive. I have included everything in the book. I have nothing more to teach you on how to overcome nail-biting! It is unnecessary! This book is already long enough for youto overcome the habit. But it will get updated with additional information. I still think I am helping you to understand, and "get the mindset" behind the scene.

My Experience Interacting With Nail-Biters. (Most of them)

So, keeping that in my mind, after publishing my book, I wanted to target a few people who are seeking to overcome nail-biting and of course; I have tried a few groups (Nail biting support groups on Facebook) to give away my book. (Brilliant idea, isn't it?) Actually NOT! It wasn't! Unfortunately, it was a really a horrible experience, mostly.

I am telling you this to make you understand and "realize "

"HOW INSECURE THE MINDSET
IS OF A NAIL-BITER? "

And absolutely, it's not their fault. What I am about to tell you didn't happen, sure that they are NOT nail-biters. Period!

Unfortunately,

Do you know that when I reached them by messaging to say that I have a free book written that I would like to give away, do they need it to try? Most of them treated me like I was a con artist who is going to steal their money; by giving away this book for absolutely FREE! Really? That's number one.

I have experienced racism, some thrown away hints that I am from a certain country which is popular with online scams, etc... That just happened. Sadly, some people just by looking at my skin color, they already put me on a trial and rejected my FREE offer. There goes number two.

Some are asking for me to show my nails to prove that I am not biting my nails anymore! Ha Ha... One guy privately messaging me. That's a good one. This is my first book. It took me eight months to put all of this information together as a newbie author, and spend thousands of dollars to make it look gorgeous. And just to give away this book for "FREE", I needed to show him my nails. How about this? If I am still biting my nails, would they believe if I just searched some images online and sent them? "Oh OK! Look at my nails!" Would they believe it? Do you know the funny part? They will. I have nothing to prove, so I let it go with a smile on my face. Number three...

There are few more horror stories I could share with you, but this will sway all the valuable information I needed you to grasp in this post chapter.

Why give energy to horror? Right?

Folks, read below very carefully.

This was "YOU" before reading this book.

So here it goes,

For the past eight months through these support groups, I had a wonderful opportunity to observe discretely, all general behaviors and insecurities of a typical nail-biter. This is a blessing for a student of the mind. Was I pitching?

"I plead guilty!"

Most of them just have the nail-biting habit, and they really looking for manicure solutions to trick the habit somehow. For some, they are happy about a product they got and stopped nail-biting for few weeks or months or so, you guessed it. They started it again, wallowing in their sad story.

The Nail Biting Princess!

I would like to call this group admin the "Nail Biting Princess" though it sounds horrible, but it is true. This is all about understanding our mindset!

She is also a heavy nail biter and made the group and according to her because it supports "each other". She occasionally shows up herself posting a video about "how much" nails she bit over the last few days after she tried some manicure products or "whatever" and saying it didn't work. And few more ladies posted few comments with sympathy saying don't worry dear! We also bit ours! Yah sure it didn't work! Have you tried this and that? I stopped biting my nails! So far, so good!

Also, another few of her fellow members heart goes to her and try to comfort her, telling "don't you worry dear, it's not only you. See, I have bitten my nails more than you... This is horrible!" So, that's it... The end of the conversation. And again and again, a few more people to show fingers and nails that are all chewed and messed up. And that's what they call "Support ". They are dwelling on this. They wallow the misery with pure "ignorance".

Few days later, another person gave life to the group with a post with some horrible photos of their fingernails and wallowing, how they hate it and the disappointment after trying a few products! Same sympathy goes to that person too! And that is what this "support group" is all about.

What did I do?

Few times I tried to convince them to use affirmations to feed opposite ideas against the habit, and they didn't realize what I was trying to say.

> "OPINIONS ARE THE CHEAPEST COMMODITIES ON EARTH! INFORMATION IS THE MOST VALUABLE!"
> NAPOLEON HILL

They are not ready to read any book to get an idea about what is going on with them. Instead, they are falling in love with a "magic" product that will stop making them biting their nails!

What I also observe about this lady, she is also having anger issues as well as insomnia. And of course other forms of OCD.

This came to my mind,

"MISERY LOVES COMPANY"

JOHN RAY (ENGLISH NATURALIST OF SEVENTEENTH CENTURY)

IN MATTHEW 15:14, JESUS SAYS, "LET THEM ALONE: THEY BE BLIND LEADERS OF THE BLIND. AND IF THE BLIND LEAD THE BLIND, BOTH SHALL FALL INTO THE DITCH."

THIS IS A NOTE TO YOURSELF!

Little to your face here, if you are an adult, and you are biting your nails, you are "NOT" a celebrity! Take some responsibility and try something that actually works. If what you are trying is not working, seek professional help! If this book is also NOT going to help, I am sorry! Seek for help! From someone who actually overcame nail-biting, or a proven professional who could help you!

Don't dwell on this with people who are in the same boat as you! They know "absolutely nothing" more than you know!

"YOU MUST KNOW IT WILL NEVER STOP UNTIL YOU TREAT THE CAUSE."

The problem is, most of them are looking for the "Gene" to give them a solution or potion to try to make it overnight.

"YOU CANNOT! YOU NEED TO HAVE A LITTLE DISCIPLINE AND PATIENCE AND KNOWLEDGE TO TREAT THE CAUSE,"

The Curse Of Dwelling On Nail Biting

Guys, now you know what is going on in this group. This is a good example to educate ourselves. You are now "aware" of it. Will they ever overcome nail-biting if things are going this way? You know the answer. Absolutely NOT!

She is making things worse here. She is making these poor people sicker! She is doing further damage not only to , but for hundreds of other followers in the group. Without her intention, of course. What do you call this?

"Ignorance,"

Where are they focusing their energy to? Along with their emotions? You guessed it. They feed more and more of the same negative thoughts to their subconscious mind. Making the habit stronger and stronger, making it harder to go away. Do they know it? Absolutely NO! Do "YOU" know it? Absolutely YES! Got my point? See how lucky you are.

"KNOWLEDGE,"

They do not understand if they could gather this information (Awareness), in this book or at least use some affirmations, or other materials. Imagine how many things could have gone so much better?

They do not understand! Because they are not "equipped" with the right information. Their mindset is not ready to accept just the right information,

They could be their own "Therapist".

So, what's all this chapter about?

We were biting our nails for so long because we were "dwelling" on the outcome. What is this outcome or the result? Damaged cuticles and nails. We keep giving more and more energy to the habit of making the habit stronger and stronger.

Every day, spend a little time to learn something new. Absorb something positive to your mind. I can't express any more, how important it is to feed positive thoughts to your subconscious mind.

My experience with other nail-biters proved my points again if you need to overcome this nasty habit, Feed polar opposite ideas against the habit (Affirmations, of course).

Gather information. Read! Get to know about nail-biting. Get "knowledge"

> "NOTHING ELSE MATTERS UNDER THE SUN"

Use time intervals. It's much better than beating yourself. But the most important thing is "Consistency ".

Don't leave a day behind. That's very important.

> HUMILIATING NAIL-BITERS OR ANY SUPPORT GROUP, OR TO EMBARRASS SOMEONE WHO IS IN ANY OF THESE SO-CALLED "SUPPORT-GROUPS" IS REALLY NOT MY INTENTION. I JUST NEED TO CONVEY THE MESSAGE THAT THESE TYPES OF SUPPORT GROUPS ARE NOT HELPING. IF FACT, SOMEONE HAS TO STAND "AGAINST" THESE GROUPS FOR THE SAKE OF OTHER POOR PEOPLE WHO ARE DESPERATE AND SEEK HELP.

THEY HAVE JOINED THESE GROUPS TO GET AN ANSWER! JUST TO SEE IF SOMETHING IS THERE TO HELP THEM OUT! I TOTALLY UNDERSTAND THE FRUSTRATION, INSECURITIES, AND INFERIORITY FEELINGS BECAUSE I HAVE BEEN THERE FOR THREE DECADES. THIS IS FOR YOUR INFORMATION ONLY. SO, IF YOU ARE ONE OF THOSE MEMBERS, I HOPE YOU PLEASE TAKE THIS POSITIVELY! I AM NOT SAYING "SORRY" AND YOU KNOW WHY…

Help yourselves! Also, help others! Get and give right information!

The next Chapter is wonderful. It's a total killer to overcome nail-biting. It's an alternative method I have recently tapped, learned and enjoyed practicing called,

HO' OPONOPONO

Are you pumped to know what it is? So, what are we waiting for? Let's turn over to the next chapter. 😊

How You Can Apply "Ho'oponopono" To Help

Cure The Nail-Biting Habit?

I will start this with my story,

Few months back I was just scrolling down my Facebook and there was an Ad that appeared of a familiar person. Of course, that is Dr. Joe Vitale from my favorite movie "The Secret".

Once again, a million times,

Thank you to "The Secret" because it started to make me look at my life in a whole another way! I meant the best possible way! It was an advertisement promoting a course.

"Ho'Oponopono,"

What was that? Just like I did after watch the movie "The Secret" out of curiosity, I just spent another fifteen minutes googling it, and of course from someone I really loved in the movie "The Secret", it turned out to be an ancient "Hawaii" meditation technique, or so you can also call it a "prayer". Dr. Joe Vitale has practiced this for a reasonable time, and he now helps people all around the world with his message about this technique called "Ho'Oponopono"

Dr. Joe Vitale was first fascinated about this technique by getting to know the legendary Ho'oponopono practitioner who cured a whole ward of criminally mental patients, not even with a single visit, but just by reading their profiles, and started healing them by healing himself using the Ho'oponopono technique.

Ho'oponopono meditation will heal you indefinitely and the fascinating thing is, you can use it to heal others as well. After I watched the introduction, I thought there is no harm in just trying it.

The feeling was abundantly refreshing, beautiful and amazing! And I can't tell you with words how I felt doing it. I am a Buddhist, and we have the meditation of "compassion". First, we have compassion to our self and after sending compassion to others. It goes on and on and I won't go any further on that. May be later.

I started doing "Ho'oponopono" more often, and I had this amazing feeling of self-love, particularity gratitude. I am still amazed at how just four simple phrases could make such a difference.

Let's talk about how to use it to cure nail-biting.

The interesting part is,

It's simple to do. But this simple technique is used to awaken the most powerful forces in the universe.

Ho'Oponopono is a meditation technique and all about compassion, love and gratitude. Particularly, when you practice it, you will feel a lot of inner peace. What else is more valuable to you? You will think from inside out. Be responsible to yourself for all the things happening outside. Which means taking responsibility for who you are, where you are now (your present circumstances), what you are doing, people and circumstances you encounter in yourself, I mean everything you can ever think of.

So let me explain, I will walk you through a simple introduction, then how to do it, and how to apply the technique for the habit.

Another Sudden Hunch

What I learned to do with this meditation was that we can apply this technique for any specific goal or a purpose. You can do this to attract money also! Then suddenly I realized that I could let people know. They can use this technique also for nail-biting, along with the techniques I have illustrated in my book!

It's been one year since I have published my book and at the time that I published my book, I had no idea about this amazing prayer.

So without further delay, here are the steps you can use the "Ho'oponopono" meditation to HELP cure the nail biting habit along with the techniques I have illustrated in the book.

There are only four very simple phrases in this meditation. As the order is not important, I will tell you the order I have been using but use in any order as you please.

> THERE ARE NO SPECIFIC POSTURES REQUIRED TO DO THIS MEDITATION. YOU CAN DO IT WHILE SITTING, STANDING, WALKING, IN BED, WHILE DRIVING AND YOU NAME IT. THIS IS A VERY SIMPLE WAY OF CLEANSING YOUR MIND, AND YOU DON'T NEED ANYONE TO TEACH YOU HOW TO DO IT. YOU DON'T NEED TO SAY ANYTHING OUT LOUD AND JUST SAY THE PHRASES IN YOUR HEAD. IT TAKES LESS THAN FIFTEEN SECONDS TO SAY ALL FOUR PHRASES. THAT'S THE BEAUTY OF IT.

The most important thing is that, when you say this out loud or in your mind, you keep the meaning of those words in mind and say them with emotions. That will only work if you don't beat yourself up to mean words every time and get emotional every time. This is a meditation technique. If you want to master a meditation, you need to practice. Everything comes with the practice. Consistency is the most important thing.

The more you do it, more you master and the sooner you will get positive results. So your dedication is similarly important.

Here goes the technique you can apply for your nail-biting habit. And apply it for any purpose. There is no harm in saying these phrases at all. It's all for good. So go crazy!

I LOVE YOU

Say "I love you" and imagine your fingers and nails. Think of them as a part of your body. See how beautiful they are and feel grateful to have them. Just don't think about anything else. Remember all of these things you need to say with feeling. It's easy. Don't worry. It will get easier as you do it. Simple, right? That's it for the first phrase.

I'M SORRY (REPENTANCE)

Again, think and imagine (It's better even if you take a little gander at your nails at this point) your fingernails and feel that you handle those nails. Feel that you need to take care of them and say sorry for any harm you caused to them because of ignorance. Remember, NOT to feel guilty. Just say sorry for your fingernails and nothing else. Got it? Cool!

Though this step could feel awkward and might resist you to hold the responsibility, don't worry. Just say sorry. Again, this will get easier as you go. Those negative thoughts of resistance are the inner "monkeys making you bite your nails." If you are feeling resistance, think of it as a good sign! It already worked! You can understand now how to apply this to any unpleasant habit you've got. If you are an alcoholic, smoker or any other drug addict, you now know how to apply it just by saying "I'm sorry".

PLEASE FORGIVE ME (ASK FORGIVENESS)

Ask for forgiveness. You'll just feel amazing! You have just said sorry and so further ask for forgiveness. This is a point testing your ego or attitude. How's the feeling when you are asking forgiveness? And from whom?

You don't need to worry about from whom you are asking for forgiveness. Just say "Please forgive me". If I am you, I would ask forgiveness from the universe. If you are a good Christian, ask forgiveness from The Lord. It doesn't matter. Ask for forgiveness. Or you can ask forgiveness from your fingernails! Why not? If you've read my book, you know, we all are connected according to the law of vibration. Ask forgiveness from your fingernails! It really doesn't matter. This is your aim.

THANK YOU (GRATITUDE)

Say "Thank You." Again, it doesn't matter to whom or what you are saying thank you for. But here is a catch, you can say thank you for your fingernails. Say thanks that you have them. Appreciate how lucky you are to have them, there are other people who don't have fingers or even arms. Say thank you that they help you eat, write, type and anything that comes to your mind.

This is the step of gratitude. Which is one of the most powerful feelings you could have.

So, what do you think? How hard this could be? If you are interested to know about starting it right away, please click this link below to a wonderful YouTube video to get an idea about how to do it. Or you can start doing along while the video is playing.

It has an amazing background music so you can focus on the phrases you are saying, and that's what I have been listening to.

Amazing Ho'oponopono meditation

https://www.youtube.com/watch?v=yDJYZXlsASg

NOTE

This is just a YouTube video. I am not getting paid for promoting this and I don't have any contacts with the video uploader. It's just an amazing Ho'oponopono meditation video that I have been using. That's it. It's simple and super easy. If you have read this seriously, I can guarantee that this will help you along with the information in my book. If you enjoyed it, appreciated it, please show your gratitude with an honest review for my book.I wish you all the very best. I am sending you blessings to get rid of the nail-biting habit once and forever!!

Share this page with anyone who's biting their nails. Make their life beautiful!

Thank you so much and I am looking forward to keeping in touch!

END FOR NOW